# New Natural Healing Encyclopedia

by
The Staff
of FC&A

FC&A Publishing
103 Clover Green
Peachtree City, GA 30269

Publisher: FC&A Publishing
Editor: Cal Beverly
Production: Laura Beverly
Cover Design: Deberah Williams
Printed and bound by Banta Company

ISBN 0-915099-25-X

# TABLE OF CONTENTS

# Cancer, General 89

# Breast Cancer 111

# Weight Loss 353

Pleasant words are like a honeycomb,
Sweetness to the soul and health to the
body.

— Proverbs 16:24


For I will restore health to you,
And your wounds I will heal,
Says the Lord

— Jeremiah 30:17a

# Introduction

*New Natural Healing Encyclopedia* is a treasure house of all the latest information about what you can do to improve your health. It tells you how to help prevent or relieve many health problems. It has been written simply to explain some of the fascinating tips that easily can be used for a naturally healthier life.

The editors and publisher of this book have been diligent in attempting to provide accurate health tips that have been confirmed by scientific research. However, this book does not constitute medical advice and should not be construed as such. We cannot guarantee the safety or effectiveness of any drug or treatment or advice mentioned. Some of these tips may not be effective for everyone. Some may work for you but not for other people. Some may work for others but not for you. The only intent of this book is to provide the consumer with easy-to-understand information.

It can be dangerous to rely on self-treatment or home remedies and neglect proven medical treatments. Medical treatment should not be ignored, but natural prevention or treatment may help, too. A good physician is the best judge of what sort of medical treatment may be needed for certain diseases.

With the rapid advances in medicine and health care, we recommend in all cases that you contact your personal physician or health care provider before taking or discontinuing any medications, or before treating yourself in any way.

Best wishes as you strive for a naturally healthier life.

# Aging and Health

## What is 'normal' aging?

Although "old age" is a state of mind, you can expect certain physiological changes to occur in your body as you age, according to a report in *Postgraduate Medicine* (85,2:213).

The following is a list of changes you may experience as you get older. (Please note that not everyone experiences these changes.)

- **Heart** — The heart's ability to work efficiently generally decreases by about one percent each year between ages 30 and 80, although regular exercise may lessen the decline. That means that normal aging will cut your heart's efficiency in half by age 80, the report indicates. "By age 80, renal (kidney) blood flow is 50 percent less and cerebral (brain) blood flow is 20 percent less than in the same person at age 30," say doctors P.E. Perlman and William Adams.

- **Lungs** — Lungs function less efficiently due to a loss of muscle tone. Smoking also reduces efficiency.
- **Kidneys** — The body becomes less efficient at flushing wastes, so certain drugs may be poisonous to the kidneys. Because the body becomes less efficient at regulating thirst, older people are also susceptible to dehydration and hypernatremia (excess sodium in the blood).
- **Digestion** — Older people have constipation more often than younger people, although the ability to absorb drugs through the intestines is unchanged. They also find it harder to swallow food because their esophagus is less efficient at moving things along.
- **Nervous system** — Impaired or confused thinking is caused by disease, not aging. But, it's natural that the brain functions more slowly, causing reflexes to slow down.
- **Immune system** — Older people are more susceptible to infections. Vaccines also have less of a beneficial effect on older folks, mainly because their immune systems have slowed down. Vaccines work by stimulating the immune system.
- **Metabolism** — Metabolism is the process by which cells release energy for maintaining the body's vital functions, such as pumping blood and regulating body temperature. Older people have more difficulty perceiving cold and are susceptible to hypothermia (body temperature dangerously below normal). Skin is less elastic and

# LIFETIME WARRANTY

## Super High-tech Video Magnetic (USA) Warrants

Your MASTER T-120 VIDEO CASSETTE, for life against all defects in material and work-manship only. This warranty applies only to the original retail purchasers and only to video cassette used according to normal practice. Defective tapes will be replaced by the sellers with proof of purchase. Such replacement shall be the sole remedy of the consumer, and there shall be no liability on the part of the manufacturer, distributor or seller for any loss or damage, direct or consequential, arising out of the use of, or inability to use, Master T-120 Video Cassette, some states do not allow the exclusion of incidental or consequential dama-ges, so the above exclusion may not apply to you. This warranty gives you specific legal rights and you may also have other rights which vary from state to state.

| A | B | C | D | E | F | G | H | I | J |
|---|---|---|---|---|---|---|---|---|---|
| 0 | 1 | 2 | 3 | 4 | 5 | 6 | 7 | 8 | 9 |
| 0 | 1 | 2 | 3 | 4 | 5 | 6 | 7 | 8 | 9 |

MASTER™

more prone to pressure sores (bedsores).

- **Thyroid gland** — The thyroid gland is located at the base of the neck and produces hormones that affect the nervous system and the digestive system. Older people are prone to hypothyroidism (decreased activity of the thyroid gland). Doctors often identify the symptoms of hypothyroidism as "failure to thrive."

Old age, by itself, should not make you feel bad, many researchers say.

## 'Failure to thrive' in the elderly

"Failure to thrive" is a murky term used by doctors to describe age-related illness in older patients. The symptoms of failure to thrive include fatigue, weakness and loss of appetite, says Dr. Richard E. Waltman. Older people may fail to thrive for a number of reasons, such as poor nutrition and stress, according to the doctor in *Senior Patient* (1,4:30).

**Depression** — Retirement, grief, financial problems or moving to a new home can cause depression, masked by pain, fatigue, weakness and loss of sleep and appetite — in other words, failure to thrive.

Doctors have difficulty helping older patients with depression because they are less likely to talk about what's bothering them than younger patients, Dr. Waltman said. The good news, however, is that once you talk to your doctor, he probably will be able to help you.

An active social life and regular exercise will give you

more energy and a happier outlook on life. Talk to your doctor about starting an exercise routine. He will advise you based on any physical limitations you might have.

**Lack of exercise** — Lack of exercise may contribute to decreased heart efficiency, muscle tone and mobility. Ironically, older people who complain of feeling tired may be told to slow down or to take it easy. That may be the worst possible advice.

"The more they rest, the more they will slow down and the worse they will feel," Dr. Waltman says. Joining an exercise group is a great way to meet new people. The activities recommended most often for older people are walking, swimming and stationary bicycling.

Always check with your doctor before beginning any exercise program.

**Poor nutrition** — A proper diet is essential for good health and "many older people simply do not eat well, especially those who live alone," Dr. Waltman said. A report in *Geriatrics* (44,8:61) points out two essential nutrients that many older people neglect.

The first is fiber, which has been shown to help prevent colon cancer by ridding the body of toxins more quickly and cleansing abnormal cells from intestinal walls.

If your diet is deficient in fiber, gradually add more. A sudden increase may cause bloating and cramps.

High-fiber foods include kidney and pinto beans, acorn squash, raspberries and prunes.

The second is calcium, which is essential in preventing osteoporosis (brittle bone disease).

Doctors recommend that you get 1,000 to 1,500 milligrams of calcium every day.

Dairy products are the best source. An eight-ounce glass of whole milk contains 291 milligrams of calcium.

**Medication problems** — If you feel poorly, and you take a number of medications prescribed by different doctors, this may be your problem, according to Dr. Waltman.

"Many older [people] take as many as 12 different medications a day…. In addition to causing side effects severe enough to justify hospital admission, medications may cause more vague symptoms of fatigue, weakness and failure to thrive," the doctor says.

**Alcohol problems** — This is not a subject many people like to talk about. But alcohol abuse does exist among older people. Too much drinking can aggravate other problems, especially those involving the liver, brain, pancreas and digestive tract.

Excessive drinking also can lead to depletion of vitamin B12, itself a serious problem. And people who consume a lot of alcohol tend to neglect their nutritional needs, leading to almost a kind of starvation.

Cut down on your drinking, if it has been a problem, says Dr. Waltman. Get help from your doctor, your local mental health association or from Alcoholics Anonymous.

**Speak your mind** — If you feel something is wrong, by all means, tell your physician. Don't wait for him to ask you about specific symptoms or stress-causing events. Says Dr. Waltman, "I have been impressed by the fact that when older patients feel something is wrong, if even vaguely, they are frequently right."

# RDA for those over 50

The tables below give the official Recommended Dietary Allowances for vitamins and minerals in amounts considered necessary for people over age 50.

The tables contain two measurement categories — (1) those vitamins and minerals that are needed in milligram amounts; and (2) those needed in much smaller microgram amounts. A milligram is one-thousandth of a gram. A microgram is one-thousandth of a milligram, or one-millionth of a gram. For comparison, it takes more than 28 grams to equal one ounce, and there are 16 ounces in one pound.

| Vitamins | Males | Females |
|----------|-------|---------|
| Vitamin A | 1000 micrograms | 800 micrograms |
| Vitamin D | 5 micrograms | 5 micrograms |
| Vitamin C | 60 milligrams | 60 milligrams |
| Folic acid | 200 micrograms | 180 micrograms |
| Niacin | 15 milligrams | 13 milligrams |
| Riboflavin | 1.4 milligrams | 1.2 milligrams |
| Thiamine | 1.2 milligrams | 1 milligram |
| Vitamin B6 | 2 milligrams | 1.6 milligrams |
| Vitamin B12 | 2 micrograms | 2 micrograms |
| Vitamin K | 80 micrograms | 65 micrograms |

| Minerals | Males | Females |
|---|---|---|
| Calcium | 800 milligrams | 800 milligrams |
| Phosphorous | 800 milligrams | 800 milligrams |
| Iodine | 150 micrograms | 150 micrograms |
| Iron | 10 milligrams | 10 milligrams |
| Magnesium | 350 milligrams | 280 milligrams |
| Selenium | 70 micrograms | 55 micrograms |
| Zinc | 15 milligrams | 12 milligrams |

People on medications or on special, restricted diets should check with their doctors before using the information above. Certain nutrients — like selenium — are dangerous in amounts only slightly above the recommended range. Check with your doctor before taking any vitamin or mineral supplements.

## Vitamin A: too little or too much can be dangerous, especially for the elderly

Vitamin A is essential for your health, but if you get too little or too much, it can be very dangerous. The RDA's for vitamin A given in Retinol equivalents (RE's) are:

| | |
|---|---|
| Infants | 375 RE |
| Children | 400-700 RE |

| Adult males | 1000 RE |
| --- | --- |
| Adult females | 800 RE |
| Pregnant females | 800 RE |
| Nursing mothers | 1300 RE |

One RE is equal to 1 microgram of vitamin A from animal sources, or 6 micrograms of vitamin A from plant sources.

Night blindness or loss of vision in near darkness is the earliest symptom of a vitamin A deficiency. A severe deficiency of vitamin A may cause xerophthalmia (dry eyes) and can lead to permanent blindness if the eye tissue becomes ulcerated, two researchers explain.

Other symptoms of vitamin A deficiency are dry, brittle hair; cracked, dry or blemished skin; itching or burning eyes; thickened eyelids; increased infections; softening of tooth enamel; loss of sense of smell; cloudy eye whites; and eventually, in extreme cases, disintegration of the eyeball, says *Vitamin Side Effects Revealed*. The lungs, digestive system and the urinary or reproductive systems may also deteriorate.

"Vitamin A deficiency is a major public health problem, particularly in industrially underdeveloped countries", the research says. "Each year an estimated one million to five million people throughout the world, usually infants and preschool children, develop vitamin A deficiency, and 100,000 to 250,000 become permanently blind." Increased cases of respiratory disease, severe diarrhea, and measles that can lead to early deaths are also associated with vitamin A deficiency.

Although vitamin A deficiency is not as common in North America or Western Europe as in poor countries, recent studies have shown that more than 20 percent of the population in those areas were receiving less than 70 percent of the RDA and could be suffering from deficiency symptoms.

Smoking, drinking alcohol, or long-term intestinal disease also can increase the body's need for vitamin A.

Natural sources of vitamin A or carotene are liver, cod liver oil, eggs, milk and dairy products, broccoli, spinach and other green, leafy vegetables, carrots, turnips and other yellow vegetables, apricots and cantaloupe. Meats naturally contain vitamin A, while plants contain a "pre-vitamin" form that the body manufactures into vitamin A.

Beta carotene is the natural raw ingredient in some foods that the body works on to turn it into full-blown vitamin A. It's a harmless nutrient — known also as pre-vitamin A — that is found in rich supply in many yellow and green vegetables.

The best part is that carotene usually is not converted into vitamin A unless the body really needs more of the vitamin. It's just burned as food energy or passes on through the body. Therefore, you can eat a lot of carotene and not suffer the same bad effect as you would from eating a lot of vitamin A. But your body normally would still get all the benefits of vitamin A without the dangers. Also, a recent study in the *Journal of Food Science* (52,4: 1022) has shown that "the carotene content of wet vegetables, either fresh or cooked, was always significantly greater than that of dried ones."

Overdoses of vitamin A can be caused by eating too much animal liver over a period of several weeks. But usually overdoses are the results of high doses of vitamin supplements, Bendich and Langseth report in the *American Journal of Clinical Nutrition* (49,2:358) — in other words, taking too many vitamin pills.

Vitamin A in the form of pills and supplements can cause more damage to the body than vitamin A and carotene consumed directly from regular food sources. That's because "dietary vitamin A is ingested throughout the day at meals, whereas supplemental vitamin A is usually taken as a single dose of preformed vitamin A in a multivitamin," the study says.

A new study from the Human Nutrition Research Center on Aging shows that "elderly people who take vitamin A supplements may be at increased risk for vitamin A overload." Adults taking repeated daily doses of around ten times the RDA have reported harmful side effects like buildup of pressure within the skull, vomiting, irritability, peeling of skin, loss of hair, dry skin and cracked lips, reports *Vitamin Side Effects Revealed* (FC&A Publishing). Megadoses can cause a toxic reaction or even, in rare cases, death.

Infants given large doses of vitamin A may suffer from itching, dehydration, muscle tremors, soft spots in the skull, and poor heart rhythm from high levels of blood calcium associated with vitamin A poisoning.

Vitamin A is fat-soluble. That means it dissolves in body fat. Because of that, it can be stored in the body for a long time, unlike water-soluble vitamins that are quickly flushed out of the body by the kidneys. The liver can store several months' supply of vitamin A (about 200,000 I.U.), so the amount of vitamin A in the body can become extremely high over many years, researchers at Tufts University report in the *American Journal of Clinical Nutrition* (49,1:112).

"Our study suggests that elderly people should limit their intake of supplemental vitamin A, particularly over the long term," warns Stephen Krasinski, who headed the research team. "Our data may also indirectly support a lowering of the RDA for vitamin A."

The good news about vitamin A overdose is that most bad symptoms will go away when the high doses are stopped. In some cases permanent damage does occur, but usually if the overdose can be diagnosed, and the additional vitamin A eliminated, the recovery will be quite rapid.

Here are some ways to avoid vitamin A overdoses:

- If you take a vitamin supplement, check the fine print on the bottle. Be sure that you never take more than the RDA for vitamin A unless your doctor specifically says it's okay.
- Do not take vitamin A supplements if you are taking cod liver oil or fish oil supplements. Both contain high levels of vitamin A. Cod liver oil or other fish oil should be used with caution, and under your doctor's supervision, because of the risk of vitamin A overdose.
- Do not take more than the RDA of vitamin A if you are elderly, unless your doctor recommends larger doses to correct a deficiency.
- If you want to supplement your body's store of vitamin A, take carotene supplements instead of vitamin A supplements.
- Do not take vitamin A supplements if you are taking isotretinoin (brand name Accutane) or etretinate (brand name Tegison). Both are prescription drugs that are made from vitamin A.
- Do not take vitamin A supplements if you are on birth

control pills, unless you also are under a doctor's supervision. Women taking birth control pills usually show an increase in levels of vitamin A in their blood of 30 to 80 percent, says *Vitamin Side Effects Revealed* (FC&A Publishing).
• Remember to always report your vitamin and mineral supplements to your doctor and, in the case of a medical emergency, the hospital staff.

## Loss of appetite and weight loss in the elderly

Loss of appetite and weight loss can lead to deteriorating health in the elderly, but doctors and families are often frustrated when they try to help. However, a recent article in *Postgraduate Medicine* (85,3:140) says that loss of appetite, known as anorexia, can usually be traced to physical or social problems and can often be alleviated.

What can trigger anorexia in the elderly? Stomach problems, prescription drugs, heart and lung diseases, dietary restrictions, isolation or even something as simple as poor-fitting dentures or a sore tooth can cause the lack of appetite and eventual weight loss, according to the study. Doctors Cynthia Olsen-Noll and Michael Bosworth of Wright State University School of Medicine co-authored the study.

Once weight loss or loss of appetite has been identified, a thorough physical exam should be given to see if a medical problem is the cause, the doctors recommend.

Some of the medical problems that the study linked to loss of appetite include the following:

- Stomach problems — peptic ulcer disease, intestinal obstruction, gallstones, stomach reflux, stomach cancer, delayed emptying of the esophagus, or spasms of the esophagus.
- Dental problems — "Absence of teeth and poor-fitting dentures can result in the avoidance of solid foods," the researchers explain. A toothache, sensitive teeth, or poor dental hygiene can also affect the appetite and the amount of food an elderly person will eat.
- Heart and lung diseases — emphysema, heart failure, and chronic bronchitis.
- Other problems — hyperthyroidism, hypothyroidism, uremia, neoplasms (unusual new tissue growth which could be cancerous) or liver problems.

Prescription and over-the-counter drugs can also affect the appetite. Levodopa (brand names Dopar and Larodopa) and digitalis (digoxin or Lanoxin) are "two drugs especially implicated in appetite suppression," the authors warn. "Oversedation by psychotropics, abuse of over-the-counter laxatives or appetite suppressants, ... thiazide diuretics," antibiotics, sedatives, narcotics and some other drugs are implicated as well.

Nutritional problems and education should not be overlooked. "Often, physicians prescribe dietary restrictions (like low-salt, high-fiber, low-fat diet) without adequately evaluating the patient's ability to understand and prepare the diet or find suitable substitutions for favorite foods," the study says.

"Older patients are more likely than younger ones to have incorrect knowledge and hold myths concerning nutrition."

Social problems can lead to appetite loss, according to the report. Since "the elderly more commonly eat for social reasons than for satisfaction," the setting and presentation of meals becomes very important. If a person lives alone, they are less likely to prepare and eat a full meal for themselves. Someone with a hearing loss may lose the enjoyment of meals because they find it difficult to talk to their companions. If the senses of taste, smell or sight are impaired, the body's natural appetite stimulants are suppressed, and such persons don't feel hungry or may not enjoy the food as much as they used to.

In an institution, a limited choice of food can cause problems. "Free choice of foods and improved socialization at mealtime improve the elderly person's overall functioning," Bosworth says.

Depression, loneliness, isolation, undiagnosed alcoholism, loss of memory, drug abuse, or anxiety can also contribute to a loss of appetite.

To overcome these problems, Olsen-Noll and Bosworth recommend a physical exam for the elderly person, reviewing and eliminating all unnecessary prescription and non-prescription drugs, improving dental care and providing better education.

They also suggest that the elderly get help in preparing special foods and allow plenty of time to eat in a comfortable social setting. The doctors also recommend an increase in physical activity when possible (such as an afternoon walk) for the elderly patient suffering from poor appetite or excessive weight loss.

# Appendicitis in the elderly may not be obvious: a telltale sign

Appendicitis in the elderly can be difficult to diagnose because they may not show the more common symptoms and signs of that illness, warns *Geriatrics* (44,4:113).

Two elderly patients at Duke University Medical Center had symptoms indicating problems in the nervous system. The nervous system symptoms included seizures, dizziness, disorientation and confusion.

Those nervous system symptoms "masked" or hid the real cause of their illness. Each of them had a severe infection of the appendix, commonly known as appendicitis. The Duke doctors call appendicitis "a common, life-threatening condition." It usually requires hospitalization and surgical removal of the infected appendix.

Even though both patients had unexplained high fever, a classic symptom of appendicitis, it took seven days for one of the patients to be accurately diagnosed.

The journal suggests that "acute appendicitis in the elderly is often difficult to diagnose" because (1) the elderly patients may also be experiencing chronic diseases; (2) they are reluctant to seek medical help; and (3) their signs and symptoms are often very different from appendicitis in a younger person.

According to the journal authors, the two signs of appendicitis to look for in the elderly are unexplained high fever and nervous system symptoms. If those two signs are present, the authors suggest that appendicitis should be considered.

## Take 'the best anti-aging vitamin' in existence — water

Water, water, everywhere, but not enough drink it.

Older folks simply don't drink enough water, especially with their medicines, says a pharmacist specializing in problems of over-age-50 patients. Maybe doctors should write prescriptions for water to make sure their older patients get enough liquid, suggests Madeline Feinberg in *Senior Patient* (1,4:26).

"All medications, including liquids, need to be taken with a half to a full glass of water," she says. "This will help the medication dissolve more quickly in the stomach and be more readily absorbed. It will also reduce any stomach irritation from the drug."

Most elderly people have to guard against drinking too little water, the article says. Older people don't get as thirsty as younger folks. Some elderly patients even try to drink less water, thinking they are "helping" their medicines. "Some people think that if pills are supposed to get rid of excess fluid, then decreasing fluid intake will be that much better!" the pharmacist writes.

Other older patients try to control loss of bladder control (incontinence) by drinking less water. Drinking less water is nearly always harmful, the article indicates, except for the few

seniors who are on doctors' orders to reduce their fluid intake.
Water has these benefits:

(1) Holds down urinary tract infections by keeping the
bladder well-flushed.
(2) Makes the best and cheapest diet drink available.
Drinking water makes you feel full with zero calories.
(3) Smooths out skin and prevents tiny wrinkles from
forming. "In fact, water is probably the best 'anti-
aging vitamin' we have for skin," the article says.

But water means water, not other beverages like coffee,
tea, soft drinks or even fruit juices, the pharmacist says.
"These (other) beverages may contain caffeine, may be high
in sugar and calories, or may interfere with drug action," the
article concludes.

# AIDS

## AIDS: a growing threat to the elderly

In just two years, there will be 27,000 cases of AIDS in people over 50, and 1,100 AIDS cases in people over 70 years of age, predicts Dr. Philip G. Weiler, director for Aging and Health at the University of California, Davis.

Weiler is worried that AIDS in the elderly is "largely an unrecognized problem" because AIDS in older people often mimics the problems of senility or Alzheimer's disease, *Geriatrics* (44,7:81) reports.

Older AIDS patients often experience loss of memory and personality changes which could easily be misdiagnosed. But Weiler points out that severe weight loss, tiredness and weakness, often will accompany the mental problems in older AIDS patients and separate them from senility patients.

"AIDS has become a diagnostic imitator. It could manifest as a psychiatric illness — for example a psychosis or depression — or simply as generalized fatigue and weight loss, perhaps mimicking cancer," says Dr. Weiler.

Why are so many elderly affected by AIDS although they haven't been considered a high-risk group? "One-fourth of all blood transfusions are in those ages 50 to 60, and you can add another 15 percent for people over age 60," he explains. "I think there is still a risk from blood transfusions that predated screening of blood donors for AIDS, which began in 1985."

AIDS typically may take many years to develop into a full-blown disease. While the diagnosis may not help the victim, such an accurate diagnosis will allow loved ones and others who give care to the victim to take appropriate precautions — precautions that might be ignored in the absence of an AIDS diagnosis.

Before finalizing a "dementia" diagnosis, doctors should check the patient's history of blood transfusions and the spouse's blood transfusion record, according to Weiler.

"The possibility of infection via sexual contact should not be ruled out," says Dr. Robert Butler, in a *Geriatrics* (44,7:21) editorial. "Physicians should not ignore or underestimate the extent of sexual involvement of people in their 50s, 60s, and older," Dr. Butler says.

"According to most estimates, 10 percent of AIDS cases are found in the over-55 population. Since this age group received more blood transfusions than any other age group, and since it may take longer to notice overt symptoms of AIDS in older persons than in younger ones, we may eventually see more cases of AIDS in the older population," according to Dr. Butler.

# AIDS through blood transfusions: how to be 100% safe

If you have surgery and need a blood transfusion, how can you be sure the donated blood is free of the deadly AIDS virus? That's a question many are asking since it was discovered that the fatal disease can be transmitted through blood transfusions.

Although every pint now undergoes strict testing to eliminate tainted blood, a small danger remains. Since March 1985, blood donated in the United States has been screened for the HIV virus, which leads to AIDS. Hepatitis B, syphilis, and another rare form of hepatitis also are screened out. But even with screening, the U.S. Surgeon General estimates that at least one pint in every 100,000 donations carries the AIDS infection and slips through to an unsuspecting recipient..

One sure way to avoid AIDS through transfusions is to donate your own blood and have it saved until you need it. A second sure way works like this: during surgery, the doctors collect blood seeping from your wounds, recycle it, and put it back in your body. These techniques are called autologous transfusion. "Autotransfusion" is another term for the same thing. This means that you give your own blood back to yourself.

Because of the AIDS crisis, many doctors are more reluctant to give blood transfusions. The National Institutes of Health have asked that all transfusions "be kept to a minimum." They definitely should be given when absolutely needed. But in some cases, the doctor will monitor the patient during the first stages of recovery and prescribe iron supplements to avoid a transfusion. "With every (regular donated blood) unit you get, the risk incrementally increases; therefore, the fewer the better," said Tibor J. Greenwalt of the University of Cincinnati in a report in *Science News*, (134:41). Dr. Greenwalt was chairman of a recent conference on transfusions at the NIH.

Still, situations may arise when you need blood, and transfusion is a medical necessity. Following are some ways you can help ensure the safety of the blood you receive.

**Autotransfusion** — Some hospitals are now capable of "recycling" blood lost during surgery, reducing the need for transfusions. Blood that was previously drained out of the body and thrown away is now being filtered, cleaned, treated, and returned to the patient. This is known as autotransfusion, because the blood is actually from the same patient.

First, the blood is suctioned out of the wound. Next, the blood is filtered to remove dangerous blood clots and any foreign materials. Blood thinners may be added. In some systems, the blood is separated in a centrifuge, and only the red cells are kept. Finally, the blood may pass through a sterile solution before it is returned to the patient.

Just approved in 1988, the Solocotrans autotransfusion system is used to help collect and recycle blood during orthopedic operations. Other systems have been in limited use for several years, but the AIDS crisis and improvements in the systems have increased their use. The Cell Saver System can be used in several types of surgery where there is usually a great loss of blood — open heart surgery, ruptured liver or spleen, ectopic (outside the uterus) pregnancy, or orthopedic operations.

Autotransfusions can be quick and cost-effective (and are usually covered by insurance companies). It takes less time to set up the equipment than it does to test for blood type and then cross-match potential blood donors from a blood bank. But some additional blood may still be needed. Doctors estimate that only one-third of the patients who use autotransfusions will not require additional blood. Two-thirds of such patients still will need donated blood.

If you are planning open heart or other surgery, find out if your hospital has a machine for autotransfusions. If you need emergency surgery, you won't have much time to make autotransfusion arrangements. To be on the safe side, check your local hospitals ahead of time.

**Pre-donating your own blood** — If you are planning elective surgery, many hospitals or blood banks will allow you to donate your own blood in advance. This blood can be stored and given back to you if it's needed during surgery.

There is a time limit. Fresh blood can be stored for only about 35 days, and you can only give a limited amount just before planned surgery. Blood can be donated, frozen for up to three years, and thawed for transfusion, but this can be extremely expensive. One pint of blood can cost $150 for freezing and $250 for thawing, not including the storage time, some officials estimate. Storage space is also limited, which often adds to the high cost per pint. Some hospitals, like Central General on Long Island, N.Y., have started hospital blood banks where patients can donate their own blood for future use.

People over age 50 or those with low blood counts may not want to give their own blood because it could weaken them and slow their recovery from surgery. Also, in cases of repeated surgery, a patient may not have enough time for recovery to pre-donate blood before the next operation.

**Pre-arranging safe donors** — Learn the blood types of yourself, your immediate family, close relatives, and best friends. Agree with each other that, in case of an emergency, each would donate blood to anyone in the group with a compatible blood type.

Keep a list of the people with your blood type, along with their telephone numbers, with you at all times. If you are in an accident or require emergency surgery, those people can be alerted. Or, if you are planning surgery, your family or friends can give a "recipient-specific" donation. The blood is tagged and kept for your use.

However, be aware that even people you know may themselves be at high risk for AIDS, but may feel pressured into giving blood for you. In that case, your safety factor would vanish. Make sure that none of these people have engaged in what the U.S. Surgeon General calls "risky behavior." This means homosexuality, injecting illegal drugs, sexual promiscuity or intimate contact with people who have done such things.

# Alcohol

## Alcohol robs your body
## of a vital nutrient

If you must drink, you'd better stop at two beers, a major new heart study suggests. More than that amount of alcohol daily may spike your blood pressure and may drain a vital nutrient, calcium, from your body, says a report by the American Heart Association. That harmful effect shows up even if you take extra calcium supplements, the study indicates.

"Our study suggests that for the average person, at more than two drinks a day, some bad things start happening physiologically," says Dr. Michael H. Criqui, co-author of the study published in *Circulation*. "Your blood pressure goes up, and you begin to lose the benefits of the calcium in your diet," Dr. Criqui says.

The study shows that non-drinkers and light drinkers who

had higher calcium intakes also had correspondingly lower blood pressures, the AHA report says.

But, the study warns, those who averaged more than two alcoholic drinks a day suffered at least two bad effects:

(1) The alcohol seemed to raise their blood pressure

(2) The drinking also seemed to prevent the blood-pressure-lowering effects of calcium.

Previous studies show that drinking alcohol apparently leads to poor absorption of calcium in the intestines, the report says. In addition, a heavier drinker passes a lot of calcium through the kidneys in urine, draining the body's stores.

Heavy drinkers sometimes have bones that appear to be "washed out" in X-ray photographs, because they lack calcium, the researcher says. That's added bad news for people at risk from osteoporosis, a bone-loss disease that strikes many women and some men over the age of 50.

You can't get around the bad effects of alcohol simply by taking more calcium every day, Dr. Criqui says. "We found that regardless of the level of calcium or potassium in the diet, alcohol still had an independent [bad] effect," says the researcher. "Alcohol seemed to be a much more powerful influence on blood pressure than either calcium or potassium."

The researcher recommends that you eliminate alcohol from your diet. Short of that, he says, you should average two or fewer alcoholic drinks a day. And because a diet rich in potassium and calcium may help reduce blood pressure, he suggests eating several servings every day of fruits and vegetables (containing potassium) and non-fat or low-fat dairy products (containing calcium).

Criqui and co-workers studied 7,011 men of Japanese descent who participated in the Honolulu Heart Study.

## Alcohol and the immune system

Heavy drinkers may be ruining more than just their liver. Excessive alcohol intake may severely damage the body's whole immune system, making it more susceptible to serious, even life-threatening infections like pneumonia, according to an editorial in the *British Medical Journal* (298,6673:543).

Heavy drinking over a period of several years may drastically decrease the number of natural "killer cells," the body's powerful defense against invading bacteria and viruses, said the report.

Heavy drinkers have much higher rates of lung infections, including tuberculosis, than other people. The drinking habit also greatly weakens the liver so that "alcoholic subjects may be at increased risk of both hepatitis and HIV (AIDS) infection," the journal said.

Undernutrition — caused by lowered intake of proteins, vitamins and sources of energy — also contributes to lowered levels of resistance to infections among heavy drinkers. Many have severe vitamin deficiencies.

# Alzheimer's Disease

## Recent research on Alzheimer's disease

Alzheimer's is a disease — always fatal — in which portions of the brain responsible for thinking, memory and routine physical functions are destroyed over a period of a few months to five years. It strikes mainly among elderly persons, and women get the disease more often than men.

Researchers in a 12-city study are looking for additional evidence that the experimental drug THA improves the ability to think and remember in patients suffering from Alzheimer's disease. Recent research suggests that THA (tetrahydroaminoacridine) slows down the abnormal loss of acetylcholine, an essential "memory" chemical made by the brain. Some researchers believe that Alzheimer's symptoms — memory loss, inability to think clearly, irrational behavior and dementia — may be caused by the decline in acetylcholine.

A second phase of the study is comparing the effectiveness of THA when taking it with and without lecithin, a natural fatty substance found in egg yolks, soybeans, corn and animal tissues.

Meanwhile, studies in recent years have shown that smokers are four times as likely as non-smokers to develop Alzheimer's disease. An obvious way to lower your risk of getting the fatal disease is to stop smoking, researchers say.

Suspicions are growing about the link between Alzheimer's and aluminum in our diet. The trace mineral has been found in abnormally high amounts in the brains of Alzheimer's victims. In such amounts, aluminum acts like a brain poison.

Some doctors are warning that aluminum in large amounts can be leached from metal utensils during cooking. *Science News* (131:73) reports that experiments in Sri Lanka suggested that cooking in aluminum cookware with water containing fluorides increases the aluminum concentration by up to 1,000 times more than cooking with water without fluorides. Most Americans routinely drink fluoridated water and use it in cooking, and many use aluminum cookware. New evidence suggests the combination may be unwise.

## Alzheimer's disease from your home tap water?

Drinking water may be harmful to your health, a new research report suggests. Aluminum levels in tap water may be linked to deadly Alzheimer's disease, one of the leading causes of senility in people from age 40 to 60, according to researchers in England.

As aluminum concentrations in ordinary drinking water increased, the rates of Alzheimer's disease among persons using that water also increased, said the report in *Lancet* (1,8629:59). In some cases, the rates increased by as much as 50 percent.

The greatest risk, they found, occurred in areas where the aluminum concentrations were greater than 0.11 milligrams (the same as 110 micrograms, or four millionths of one ounce) per liter of water. (One liter is equal to about one and one-half quarts.) Below 0.01 milligrams (10 micrograms) aluminum per liter, the researchers found, there seemed to be no added risks of getting Alzheimer's disease.

Aluminum sulfate, or alum, is commonly used by water systems during the treatment process, the report said. The chemical is added at the water plant as a coagulant to make suspended solids settle out of the liquid.

The amount of aluminum added varies from plant to plant, within certain limits, depending on the amount of solid materials present in the raw water being treated. In many cases, increased amounts of aluminum added to the raw water means that technicians have to use less chlorine to purify the water later in the treatment process.

While much of the added aluminum is removed before the water is pumped to homes and schools, some aluminum remains dissolved in the treated water and is consumed by water users, the report said. Higher levels of aluminum in untreated water also occur naturally in some geographic locations because of mineral deposits in the ground.

For comparison, a recent chemical analysis of water

treated by the Atlanta, Ga., water system showed that the after-treatment aluminum level was 0.06 milligrams (60 micrograms) per liter. The British study indicated that, at that level, Alzheimer's disease rates increased by about 40 percent in the areas studied in England and Wales.

Aluminum is not among the "toxic" chemicals for which many U.S. water systems routinely test their water supplies and for which maximum limits are set. For example, there are no current standards or limits on aluminum concentration for Georgia water systems. The 12-nation European Economic Community currently permits water aluminum concentrations up to 0.2 milligrams (200 micrograms) per liter, according to an editorial in the same issue of *Lancet*.

The researchers were concerned that the water treatment process may add to the already high levels of aluminum consumption in most Western countries. In Britain, for example, they estimated that an adult consumes an average of five to 10 milligrams of aluminum each day, occurring naturally in food. But, researchers say, only a small portion of that is actually absorbed by the body internally.

Aluminum-based preservatives in food may add another 50 milligrams (50,000 micrograms) daily. An adult American may get that much or more of the chemical, especially since many people regularly take aluminum-based antacids for heartburn and upset stomach.

While much of that aluminum passes through the body without being absorbed, the British researchers were concerned that water aluminum is much more "bioavailable." That means it is more easily absorbed during its passage through the digestive system. They recommended that water plants use as little aluminum as possible during the treatment process to cut down on the long-term accumulation of the chemical in humans.

Although aluminum is considered a "trace element" (*Taber's Cyclopedic Medical Dictionary*, 16th edition, 1989: p.1885) and is found in minute quantities in food, water and living tissues, the body does not require aluminum for any metabolic processes. In fact, aluminum is increasingly under suspicion as a potent brain poison.

Autopsies have revealed abnormally high amounts of aluminum in characteristic "tangles" of diseased tissue in brains of persons who died with Alzheimer's disease. More suspicions were raised in the mid-1970s when young patients undergoing dialysis treatment for kidney disease developed symptoms of senility. Doctors found that aluminum in the water used in the treatment caused the rapidly developing senility. When they lowered the aluminum below 0.03 milligrams (30 micrograms) per liter, the senility symptoms were quickly reversed, and the patients returned to normal mental states.

Residents of the island of Guam, where the water is high in aluminum and low in calcium and magnesium, have more cases of amyotrophic lateral sclerosis, also known as Lou Gehrig's disease. That disease also causes senility and leads to death. It is very similar to Alzheimer's disease, especially in the abnormally high amounts of aluminum found in the brain tissue at autopsy.

The British researchers indicated that they are convinced of a strong relationship between long-term aluminum consumption and increased risks of getting Alzheimer's disease.

"This survey, conducted in 88 county districts within England and Wales, shows that rates of Alzheimer's disease in people under the age of 70 years are related to the average aluminum concentrations present in drinking water supplies over the previous decade," the report said. "A positive relation between rates of Alzheimer's disease and water aluminum concentrations was present whichever way the data were analyzed."

Readers may want to call their local water system to find out the concentration of aluminum in drinking water. If it is above 0.01 milligrams (10 micrograms) per liter, some home filtering system may be warranted. In addition, water systems might be encouraged to use less aluminum in the treatment process, pending further scientific study of the potential threat of long-term aluminum ingestion.

# Arthritis

## Weapons for fighting arthritis

Arthritis, in one of its more than 100 forms, afflicts millions of Americans. A lot of sufferers want answers about what's causing the pain and what can be done to treat it. Here are a few questions and answers:

**Q. Arthritis — what is it?**

**A.** The term means "inflammation of a joint." There are more than 100 different diseases that are considered forms of arthritis. All of them attack joints and connective tissues in the body. But each form has different symptoms, and each must be treated differently.

The most common form is osteoarthritis, affecting 16 million Americans. This type happens when the elastic surfaces at the end of bones — called cartilage — begin deteriorating. Osteoarthritis usually strikes people over 60, affecting mostly joints in the feet, fingers, hips and knees. It usually hits only a few joints at any one time.

Next most common is rheumatoid arthritis. In this disease, the film-like membrane surrounding a joint becomes inflamed, eventually leading to destruction of the joint itself. Rheumatoid arthritis strikes people of various ages and can affect many joints at once. It can even cause problems with other organs like the eyes, lungs, blood vessels and skin.

Other forms include spinal arthritis (known medically as ankylosing spondylitis), lupus, gout, scleroderma and juvenile arthritis, according to *Arthritis Today* (3,3:22).

**Q. What causes arthritis?**

**A.** Although exact causes are still uncertain, scientists are beginning to think that some people may inherit the tendency to get arthritis, especially the rheumatoid variety, according to the Arthritis Foundation.

Several forms also seem to be triggered by certain kinds of infections. For example, some kinds of diseases caused by tick bites can lead to arthritis-like inflammations in the joints. But "triggers" are not the same things as "causes."

**Q. What can be done to treat arthritis?**

**A.** There is no known cure. However, the pain and crippling of arthritis usually can be controlled, especially if the disease is caught early. Control measures include medicines, diet, exercise, rest, protection of the affected joints and, sometimes, surgery, including replacement of whole joints with artificial materials.

Many people seem to believe that arthritis is a natural result of growing old and think that arthritis isn't harmful, so they treat themselves rather than going to a doctor. However, since there are several different types of arthritis, and because of the high death-rate in rheumatoid arthritis, a doctor should always be consulted.

Early and aggressive treatment of rheumatoid arthritis is very important. British researchers have found that waiting too long to treat rheumatoid arthritis can be fatal. According to a 25-year study by the Royal National Hospital for Rheumatic Diseases in Bath, England, one-third of people with rheumatoid arthritis died because of arthritis-related problems.

"People really do die from arthritis," cautioned Dr. Theodore Pincus of Vanderbilt University in Nashville. Furthermore, medical treatment within the first six months of rheumatoid arthritis also can prevent irreversible damage to the joints and cartilage, as well as lowering the death rate, the researchers concluded.

Treatment varies, depending on the patient and the specific type of arthritis.

**Q. What medicines are used to treat arthritis?**

**A.** There are three categories of drugs used to control arthritis.

    (1) The main type fights inflammation, the major source of arthritis pain. Among these are the nonsteroidal anti-inflammatory drugs (known as NSAIDs) and the corticosteroids. Aspirin is the best-known of the NSAIDs and probably is used more than any other single medicine to treat arthritis, says *Arthritis Today*.

    (2) Another category of drugs acts to slow down the disease process, which, untreated, leads to destruction of the affected joint. This second class of drugs includes gold compounds, penicillamine, methotrexate

and anti-malarial drugs. All these are very powerful and have some serious side effects.

(3) The drugs of last resort are extremely powerful immunosuppressives. That means they put a damper on the body's own self-defense system. They may halt the disease's progress, but the potential side effects are severe.

**Q. What are some other treatments?**

**A.** The Arthritis Foundation says sufferers get some relief from both heat and cold therapies. "Cold temporarily deadens nerves that carry pain and also reduces swelling and inflammation," according to the report in *Arthritis Today.* "We really don't know why heat works. It does increase circulation in the affected area ... One popular technique for pain relief is a contrast bath ... alternating use of heat and cold."

**Q. What about diet and other natural means?**

**A.** Aerobic exercise is recommended for people who have mild or moderate forms of arthritis. Studies have shown that low-intensity exercise like fast walking or golfing actually can reduce joint pain in patients with rheumatoid and osteoarthritis, according to the medical journal *Physician and Sportsmedicine* (17,2:128).

In gouty arthritis, diet may play a major role in prevention of the painful attacks.

If rheumatoid arthritis is suspected, fish oil may reduce the painful symptoms, says Dr. Edward Harris, chairman of medicine at Stanford University. This is especially effective if treatment with the oil is supplemented with daily aspirin, Harris told *Medical World News.*

Doctors recommend getting the essential ingredients in

fish oil—the omega-3 fatty acids—by eating cold-water fish rather than by taking fish oil capsules. High levels of these beneficial oils are found naturally in all cold-water fish. Increase your intake of trout, salmon, mackerel, or cod. Packaged fish oil supplements, available at the store, could cause other problems, such as reducing the ability of your blood to clot. For that reason, most doctors believe the supplements should be used with caution.

## Some current research about arthritis treatment

You may be able to reach into your kitchen spice cabinet for relief from the pain and inflammation of rheumatoid arthritis. Arthritis patients reported "significant relief" from pain after taking less than a tablespoonful of ginger every day for three months, reports Dr. Krishna C. Srivastava of the Institute of Odense in Denmark. Long known as a folk remedy for various ailments, ginger now is being studied in medical trials to determine its usefulness as an arthritis medicine.

The arthritis patients took ginger in two ways: either about five grams a day of fresh ginger root, or from a half-gram to 1.5 grams daily of ginger powder. All reported that "they were able to move around better and had less swelling and morning stiffness after taking the spice," says *Medical Tribune* (30,18:16). No side effects were reported.

Another potential medicine comes from China and has been used there for centuries as a folk remedy. Researchers are planning large-scale trials of an extract from an herb known as Tripterygium wilfordii hook.

The Chinese extract "achieved a 90 percent reduction in pain and other typical RA symptoms in 30 patients who were treated for 12 weeks," according to the *Tribune* report. Control patients given a placebo (a harmless fake medicine) recorded less than a fourth as much relief. The main side effects were skin rash in half the patients and mild diarrhea in about a fifth.

Still another natural source of arthritis help is showing up in bark extracts from an Indian tree known as Dysoxylum binectariferum. The extract, known as rohitukine, has been shown to cut inflammation and decrease some bad effects of the body's own immune system turning against itself, according to Dr. A.N. Dohadwalla in Bombay. Even high dosages produced no bad side effects in animal tests, the doctor says.

In addition, possible arthritis help may come from deposits of decaying vegetation. A plant extract tested recently comes from some rich peat bogs in Poland. Peat is a soft forerunner of coal.

The refined product seems to cut down on the autoimmune response that, in rheumatoid arthritis, points the body's anti-disease weapons at the body tissues themselves.

## Arthritis, a sleep-robber?

Eight out of 10 people with rheumatoid arthritis report that they often feel very tired during the day. Doctors usually say that daytime fatigue is just part of the suffering that rheumatoid arthritis patients have to learn to put up with. Many doctors see tiredness as a measure of the disease's activity and of drug therapy to fight arthritis.

But a new study in *Arthritis and Rheumatism* (32,8:974) suggests that many cases of such fatigue may be due to sleep disturbances, rather than an organic side effect of the disease itself. Doctors at the Minnesota Regional Sleep Disorders Center studied 16 patients with chronic, active rheumatoid arthritis, but who were otherwise healthy. The youngest was 54; the oldest, 71. They found no "sleep deprivation" as such.

The doctors were surprised, however, to find that all 16 rheumatoid arthritis patients thrashed their arms and legs much more than "normal" sleepers. Perhaps more significantly, all 16 awoke frequently throughout the night, many times more than non-arthritic patients, the report indicates.

Based on brain-wave readings, the rheumatoid arthritis patients averaged waking up and dozing off an amazing 46 times per hour, "which permitted only 1.3-minute sleep periods," the report says. More than 10 of those awakening periods lasted more than a minute each, the study says. That's two to three times the sleep-arousal rate of a group of non-arthritic 75-year-olds in another study.

Perhaps even more amazing, none of the 16 realized the next day how badly he had slept. All remembered waking up only about half the times they actually did, as measured objectively by the researchers on their instruments. More than half the group had two other sleep disorders affecting the depth of their sleep and the length of time they spent in bed. Interestingly, not one of the 16 blamed waking up on joint pain.

The doctors avoided trying to limit the effects of medicines on the tests. They reasoned that rheumatoid arthritis patients generally take medicines, and that must be factored in. Nine of the patients were taking prednisone, but the seven who were not taking that medicine had the same sleep problems. None was taking any kind of sleeping pill. One was taking amitriptyline, and one was on imipramine, both only occasional low doses.

"These striking abnormalities of sleep" may cause excessive daytime sleepiness in rheumatoid arthritis patients, the researchers conclude, "and may play a role in early-onset fatigue." The implication from this study is that this rheumatoid arthritis "symptom" may be a separate illness.

Until now, doctors have treated the arthritis but generally have not tried to fight the "accompanying" fatigue. Now, they may want to start treating the tiredness itself, separate from the arthritis.

## Fibromyalgia: an arthritis-like disease

Fibromyalgia is a condition affecting the muscles that causes intense, widespread pain at various "tender points" throughout the body. Other symptoms include anxiety, fatigue, headache, disturbed sleep, bowel problems and numbness or tingling sensations. Fibromyalgia affects an estimated five percent of Americans, mostly women, and is often mistaken as an inevitable side effect of arthritis. The disease, once called fibrosis, is kin to arthritis, and people with arthritis also can suffer from fibromyalgia at the same time.

Doctors still don't know what causes it. They point out that the symptoms are very similar to those of chronic fatigue syndrome. That leads some to speculate that stress, anxiety, depression and emotional upsets may trigger the condition or make it worse. Research centers on finding out whether these factors cause the disease or result from the disease. Other doctors think that the disease may be caused by some kind of virus.

No X-ray or laboratory test yet exists that can identify the condition. Because of that, over the years, fibromyalgia patients have been told by doctors that the pain is "all in their heads." However, doctors are finally getting a grip on diagnosing this hard-to-pin-down disease.

Recently, rheumatologists have identified several specific tender points to distinguish fibromyalgia from other painful rheumatic conditions like osteoarthritis. Doctors now can test a patient's pain level just by pressing those areas with their hands. That eliminates the need for expensive blood tests and X-rays.

You can tell whether you have the disease by touch. If you feel pain at 11 out of 18 touch points, you could be suffering from fibromyalgia, the report indicates. "Tenderness in at least 11 of 18 specified sites on the body, accompanied by widespread pain, identifies the syndrome and distinguishes it from other ... disorders," says Dr. Frederick Wolfe, chairman of the Multicenter Fibromyalgia Criteria Study.

The tender points that you and your doctor can look for are as follows:

- **Neck** — four points: one point on each side of the larynx (voice box). Also, on the back of the neck, one spot on either side of the spinal column at about the midway point on the neck.
- **Back** — four points: one on the outside of each shoulder blade, and one point near the middle of the shoulders at an outward angle from the shoulder blade.
- **Hips** — four points: one at the top of each buttock, and one point on the lower outside of each hip.
- **Chest** — two points: one spot on each side of the breastbone at the second rib, just below the collarbone.
- **Legs** — two points: one site on the inside of each knee.
- **Arms** — two points: one spot on the inside of each elbow.

Though there is still no cure for fibromyalgia, doctors are discovering some treatments for it, according to reports in *Arthritis Today* (3,3:50) and *Medical World News* (30,11:10).

- You can put ice packs or heating pads on the painful areas. Sometimes a combination of both these approaches can help.
- You can do some aerobic exercises that work on the muscle areas giving you pain.
- You can do certain stretching exercises that may provide some relief.
- You can stand erect and sit properly. Poor posture is known to aggravate the condition.
- You can learn several stress reducing techniques, such as meditation, reading the Bible, etc.

Check with your doctor first about these and other natural ways you can ease the pain. Your doctor also may want to prescribe sleeping pills and some muscle relaxers. Treatment is tailored to the patient, depending on how badly she hurts and where.

For more information about fibromyalgia and what you can do to fight its painful effects, contact your local Arthritis Foundation chapter.

# Asthma

## Soybean dust linked to
## severe asthma attacks

If you suffer from asthma attacks, the villain causing your distress may be as near as your pantry. Epidemics among dockworkers and residents living near the docks in Barcelona and Cartagena, Spain have led researchers to identify a new asthma trigger: soybean dust, according to reports in *The Lancet* (2,8662:538) and *The New England Journal of Medicine* (320,17:1097).

Soybeans are a member of the legume family, which includes peas and beans. A common U.S. farm crop, soybeans are high in protein and are used in many commercially prepared foods. Soy products include soy flour and oil, both of which are used in many food products, from margarine to fillers in canned and frozen meat products.

According to the reports, "extracts of the bean can cause

an immediate allergic response." During one epidemic, researchers found that 64 of 84 adults were allergic to soybean products. For some reason, children under age 14 were not affected. In another epidemic, 65 patients were sent to the hospital with acute asthma. One died, and nine others needed a respirator to help them breathe.

Experts have known for some time that air pollution and thunderstorms, which stir up a lot of dust, cause asthma epidemics. But, the reports say, the weather was not a factor in the 13 epidemics in Barcelona. On each asthma epidemic day, however, dockworkers were unloading soybeans. No epidemics were reported on days when soybeans were not unloaded.

Researchers point out that the increasing popularity of soybean products may lead to asthma epidemics in other parts of the world. If you are experiencing unexplained breathing difficulties or allergies, ask your doctor to test you for sensitivity to soy products.

## New research about asthma and allergies

All asthma is caused by allergies, according to a new study by researchers at the University of Arizona. "These findings challenge the concept that there are basic differences between so-called allergic ("extrinsic") and nonallergic ("intrinsic") forms of asthma", reports Dr. Benjamin Burrows in the *New England Journal of Medicine* (320:271-7).

In the new study, doctors found that the prevalence of asthma was related to the level of the serum immunoglobulin (IgE). "And no asthma was present in the 177 subjects with the lowest IgE levels for their age and sex," they report. IgE is the antibody that causes immune system response in the body. Excessive amounts of that antibody occur during allergic reactions.

More than 2,600 volunteers with asthma or allergic rhinitis were compared by levels of serum IgE and allergic reactions to skin tests. Asthma was found in direct correlation with the IgE levels and the skin test seemed to have no effect. However, people with allergic rhinitis "appeared to be associated primarily with skin-test reactions to common aeroallergens" and the IgE levels were insignificant, the doctors said. Aeroallergens are airborne triggers of allergic reactions.

"We conclude that asthma is almost always associated with some type of IgE-related reaction and therefore has an allergic basis," the report states.

Since 1918, doctors have believed that some asthma is caused by allergies to dust, molds, pollens, animal danders and other airborne particles. But if the asthma is triggered by emotional factors, infection or irritants, it is classed as nonallergic. According to *The Merck Manual*, about 10-20 percent of adults have allergic asthma, 30-50 percent have nonallergic asthma and some seem to have allergic and nonallergic responses.

Now, this belief will have to be reevaluated.

# Blood Pressure

## The facts about high blood pressure

High blood pressure is the major risk factor for stroke and one of the major risk factors for heart attacks and cardiovascular problems as well as kidney failure. Although high blood pressure may be partly hereditary, several "environmental" factors increase the likelihood you may get it. They include stress, obesity, a sedentary lifestyle, low potassium intake and too much fat, salt and alcohol.

Many Americans take medication to control high blood pressure. Although medication does help, researchers are concerned about the effects of long-term use—especially for people whose blood pressure is just above normal—and are exploring ways to lower it naturally through diet and exercise.

If you have high-normal blood pressure, exercising, losing weight and watching salt and alcohol intake can help bring your blood pressure under control, according to a study in the *Journal of the American Medical Association* (262,13:1801).

Nutritionists advise that you develop a taste for less salty foods and for more fruits and vegetables, especially in their raw forms. They provide a good source of potassium, which helps to keep your blood pressure in line, as well as to prevent strokes. Losing weight also seems to be a big factor in lowering your blood pressure.

## Before you treat high blood pressure, read this

Blood pressure readings taken at home are more accurate than readings taken at a doctor's office when it comes to predicting heart disease, a new study has discovered. This means that if a doctor only relies on the office readings, many people could be incorrectly treated for mild high blood pressure.

Although doctors have known for almost 50 years that a trip to the physician or the hospital can cause an inflated blood pressure reading—often called "white coat hypertension,"—doctors did not know if these people were at higher risk for heart disease than people with normal readings. Higher office readings are labeled "white coat hypertension" because blood pressure sometimes rises when patients feel stressed by a visit to the doctor. According to the study, 10 to 20 percent of all people with mild high blood pressure may suffer from "white coat hypertension".

However, a report just published in the *Journal of the American Medical Association* (261:873) showed that people with "white coat hypertension" did not have the heart damage associated with high blood pressure — an enlarged heart and reduced heart function.

Sustained and untreated high blood pressure can damage the heart, arteries, kidneys, brain, and eyes. People with uncontrolled high blood pressure have seven times more strokes, four times as much congestive heart failure and three times as much coronary heart disease as people with normal blood pressure.

In the study at the University of Connecticut, people with high office readings but normal readings at home were compared to two groups — one that had high blood pressure and one that had normal blood pressure. The office and home blood pressure readings of all three groups were recorded. The size and capacity of their hearts were evaluated at rest and during exercise. People with "white coat hypertension" were found to have normal heart function and no physical signs of true high blood pressure.

The researchers suggest that since there is no apparent heart damage, people with "white coat hypertension" do not have high blood pressure. To avoid unnecessary treatment, people with mild high blood pressure could be monitored at home before any drug treatment is started. Portable units are available to take and record blood pressure at regular intervals. Patients wear the monitors throughout the day and keep a record of their physical activities. Later, the doctor compares the blood pressure readings to the corresponding physical activities.

Also, many doctors are now encouraging their patients with high blood pressure to monitor their own levels manually. Patients are taught to use their own stethoscopes and cuffs and record their readings at home. They bring their "blood pressure diary" to each checkup by the doctor. This way, the doctor can evaluate the patient based on their normal daily blood pressure, rather than on an inflated blood pressure reading taken during an occasional, but stressful, visit to the doctor's office.

Since about 45 million Americans are estimated to have "mild" high blood pressure, and up to 20 percent of those are estimated to suffer from "white coat hypertension," over eight million Americans could be affected by these findings.

## New way to measure blood pressure

Stethoscopes and blood pressure cuffs may turn out to be an "old-fashioned" way to measure blood pressure, according to a Cardiovascular Research Report of the American Heart Association.

Instead, blood waves are key elements of a new, non-invasive method of recording blood pressure, developed at the Cardiovascular Center of Cornell University Medical College. This method, which records sounds made by pulsing blood and transforms them into a printed waveform graph, is more reliable and more accurate than traditional techniques, the scientists reported in *Circulation*.

Dr. Seymour G. Blank, a physiologist/engineer who leads

the research team, said the sound of the blood flowing in the arteries is recorded "using a specially designed microphone quite similar to those in personal tape recorders and telephones." The microphone is placed over the arm and captures sounds in the arteries made as the blood-pressure cuff is deflated. The sounds are transformed into continuous waves plotted on a graph, giving doctors much more information than the two numbers currently used to evaluate blood pressure.

As the sound-wave frequencies change, three distinct patterns or waveforms emerge. Scientists tagged them K1, K2 and K3 — the "K" is for the Russian physician Nikolai Korotkoff, developer of the currently used sound-evaluation method of measuring blood pressure. The systolic and diastolic blood pressures are recorded in wave K2, the researchers found. The K3 wave measures pressures in arteries that carry blood away from the heart.

Listening through a stethoscope while a blood-pressure cuff is inflated over the arm, Korotkoff's method is now the standard way to measure blood pressure. It is taken in two readings: for example, 120/80, and normally spoken of as "120 over 80." The first number refers to systolic pressure, the pressure that is produced as the heart contracts to pump blood out into the body. The second number refers to diastolic pressure, the pressure that remains in the blood vessels as the heart relaxes to allow for the flow of blood into its pumping chambers.

"That method is adequate in many patients," said Dr. Franco B. Mueller, assistant professor of medicine and co-author of the study. "However, it doesn't always work well in persons who are obese, children, dehydrated patients and those who are seriously ill in the intensive care unit." In some critically ill people, a catheter is inserted into a blood vessel to monitor blood pressure. But using a catheter increases the risk of infection and bleeding. The sensitive wave technique should enable more accurate monitoring of blood pressure in difficult situations without catheterization, he explained.

Recorded waves of blood pressure will also be more reliable, Mueller suggested. "Two people don't hear exactly the same thing ... when checking blood pressure. The waveforms are something objective that can be measured."

A similar method, which would eliminate the cuff but makes use of the printed waves, is being developed at the Technion-Israel Institute of Technology in Haifa, Israel. Their experimental monitor uses a small wrist band that is more comfortable than a cuff, according to its developers. And the reading will be taken in just one second, compared to more than a minute needed for current measurement.

## Important new risk factor for blood pressure deaths

Measuring a common waste product from your body may be the best early warning sign yet discovered to signal your risk of death from high blood pressure. Researchers have discovered that a blood test frequently performed during routine medical examinations may be a highly accurate predictor of fatality in patients with hypertension.

More than 50 percent of people with a combination of high blood pressure and high levels of a substance called creatinine in the blood will die within eight years, the report says.

Researchers analyzed data from a massive study involving 14 U.S. medical schools. Among the 10,940 high blood pressure patients enrolled in the study, a high level — 2.5 milligrams per deciliter or more — of a substance called creatinine in their blood serum was associated with a surprisingly high death rate, according to a report in *Hypertension* (13,1:1).

"These data suggest that in patients with high blood pressure and a serum creatinine level equal to or greater than 2.5, more than 50 percent will die within eight years," says Dr. Neil B. Shulman, a principal investigator in the study.

Beginning at a serum creatinine level of 1.2, there was a noticeable, continuous increase in risk of death at increasing levels of creatinine, Shulman says. A normal creatinine range is usually considered to be between 0.7 and 1.5 milligrams per deciliter, he adds. It's not that creatinine by itself causes anything bad to happen. High levels of it just serve like a smoke detector's buzzer, warning that something bad is going on in the body.

Creatinine is a waste product of metabolic processes in muscle cells, like smoke from a fire, explains Shulman, associate professor of medicine at Emory University in Atlanta. Normally, the kidneys filter creatinine out of the blood. For that reason, high levels of creatinine in the blood also may indicate kidney problems. But the patients with high creatinine levels tended to die of heart disease and stroke, not of kidney disease, the scientists found. "We don't know why the hearts and brains of these patients with kidney dysfunction are so vulnerable to heart attacks and stroke," Shulman says.

The new finding is important, he adds, because it might lead to new approaches to preventing the complications of high blood pressure, which include heart attack and stroke. According to Shulman, the study indicates that high blood levels of creatinine should be recognized as a risk "marker" for stroke and heart attack.

An abnormal electrocardiogram (ECG) or an enlarged heart are other risk "markers." Conventional risk factors include cigarette smoking, elevated serum cholesterol and high blood pressure.

"I think our finding will be valuable both to the researchers who are trying to unravel the mysteries of high blood pressure and to the practicing physicians who need to identify which patients deserve special attention," Shulman says. Patients with high creatinine levels are in such a "risky situation" that physicians should work hard to help them reduce their risk factors for heart attack and stroke, he says.

## A plan to prevent high blood pressure naturally

If you are prone to high blood pressure, are you destined to be forced to take powerful drugs to fight the disease? The answer is, maybe not. You may have a natural option to prevent high blood pressure from ever developing, say eight researchers at Northwestern University Medical School in

Chicago.

"Results indicate that even a moderate reduction in risk factors for hypertension among hypertension-prone individuals contributes to the primary prevention of the disease," the report says. (Hypertension is the scientific name for high blood pressure.)

You may be able to cut your risk of developing high blood pressure by following these same moderate changes in lifestyle, the scientists indicate in a report in the *Journal of the American Medical Association* (262,13:1801).

The researchers studied 201 men and women who were slightly overweight, ate salty foods, smoked, downed several alcoholic drinks a day, and rarely exercised. All of them had blood pressure in the "high-normal" range. That means a diastolic (lower number) pressure of from 80 to 99 mm Hg. But, otherwise, they all were healthy.

These prime candidates for high blood pressure agreed to work on better nutrition and to shoot for four goals:

(1) lose at least 10 pounds,
(2) reduce daily salt intake to less than one-tenth of an ounce,
(3) cut back to no more than two alcoholic drinks a day, and
(4) exercise for 30 minutes three times a week.

Smokers were advised to kick the habit. The researchers encouraged the study participants to stick to a "fat-modified American Heart Association-type diet."

For five years, the participants — ranging in age from 30

to 44 — kept food diaries, visited with the doctors regularly, were given blood and urine tests, and had their blood pressures checked periodically. Three-quarters of them exercised faithfully, mostly walking, jogging and bicycling. One out of four met the weight-loss goal, but fewer than two in 10 reduced salt intakes. All said they averaged no more than two drinks a day. They cut their daily calorie intake by an average of 800 calories, a drop of 30 percent. They cut back modestly on saturated fat and cholesterol.

During the same period, doctors kept track of another, similar group that took no special dietary, weight-loss or exercise measures — in other words, just everyday folks who continued to eat, drink and do what they pleased.

After five years, the researchers found that the "do-as-you-please" group had double the rate of high blood pressure as the study group. The nutritional approach also helped even those in the study group who did develop high blood pressure by delaying its onset for a year or more in most cases. Those who lost the most weight experienced the most benefits, the researchers report. On the negative side, smokers were nearly four times as likely to develop high blood pressure as non-smokers, the report indicates.

One in five people in the "do-as-you-please" group developed high blood pressure during the five-year trial, compared with one in 11 in the nutrition study group. That proved true even though most in the study group did not reach their original goals. Just the emphasis on nutrition seemed to help a lot.

Such modest changes in lifestyle could slash the risks of heart disease and stroke in 1 million people with high-normal blood pressure over the next five years, the researchers believe. "Savings in numbers of cases among older persons would enlarge this potential even further," the report says. The researchers recommend that doctors start aiming for "primary prevention [of high blood pressure] by safe nutritional-hygenic means" in addition to prescribing drugs to fight the disease.

## New study confirms that blood pressure can be lowered naturally

Blood pressure can be lowered without drugs, a new four-year study by the University of Minnesota confirms. The researchers found that even people with mild high blood pressure, who had been taking prescription drugs, could maintain lower blood pressure without drugs by losing weight, reducing salt, and reducing alcohol.

"Drugs have saved the lives of many people with high blood pressure," explained Dr. Richard H. Grimm, Jr. who led the study. "But in recent years, the medical community has been more and more concerned about the potential adverse side effects of drugs and the cost of drugs."

In the study, 189 men who had mild high blood pressure (those with controlled diastolic blood pressure less than 90 mm/Hg) were divided into three groups. The first group stopped taking prescription drugs and received nutritional counseling. "They were instructed in weight control, dietary sodium reduction and alcohol reduction," Grimm explained. The second group discontinued drug therapy but did not receive any nutritional counseling. Group three continued on their prescription drug regimen.

"Four years after the study began, almost 40 percent of group one participants remained off drugs with normal blood pressures," the researchers reported. But 95 percent of groups two and three had to be returned to drug therapy.

The non-drug, nutrition group lost an average of 5 to 10 pounds and kept the weight off during the four years. Their salt intake was reduced by 36 percent, and the amount of alcohol they consumed was also reduced. However, the other groups gained weight and showed no change in their salt and alcohol intakes.

Group one also had improved levels of cholesterol, potassium and uric acid in the blood, an unexpected but pleasant side effect, the doctors noted. "The promising non-drug treatments include weight control, dietary sodium reduction, alcohol reduction, and programs to increase physical activity in people with mild high blood pressure," Grimm reported.

Grimm is also heading another study, called the Treatment of Mild Hypertension Study, sponsored by the National Heart, Lung and Blood Institute. Grimm hopes the study will show the following:

(1) if nutrition therapy combined with drug therapy will lower the death rate from high blood pressure,

(2) if lowering mild blood pressure will prevent coronary heart disease, and

(3) how different blood pressure drugs affect life expectancy.

"The Treatment of Mild Hypertension Study has enormous

social and economic implications because an estimated 45 million Americans have 'mild' hypertension," Grimm warned. "Careful evaluations of these treatments are crucial because the 1988 report of the National Joint Committee of the Detection and Treatment of High Blood Pressure recommends initial non-drug therapy for 'mild' hypertension, and has broadened initial drug therapy to include ACE inhibitors and calcium channel blockers." These drugs and other new high blood pressure drugs "have direct costs 5 to 15 times higher than generic thiazide diuretics," Grimm explained.

"Approximately 60 million Americans — about 25 percent of the adult population — have high blood pressure", Grimm reports. "The medical costs of hypertension are estimated about $10 billion annually ... approximately 75 million patient visits to primary-care physicians for high blood pressure treatment each year."

## Learning to like a low-salt diet

A low-sodium diet is one of the basic, natural ways to lower high blood pressure, but many people are hesitant because they think that a salt-free diet is bland. However, researchers at the University of Minnesota discovered that your desire for salt and your taste changes when you start a low-salt diet.

"The study was initiated because many participants in earlier studies reported that once they were on a low-sodium diet, many foods that had been acceptable were now 'too salty' or even unpleasant," Dr. Richard Grimm recently announced.

Participants on a low-salt diet compared salted crackers at regular intervals. "The highest sodium content crackers were rated more salty and less pleasant," Grimm said. "The level of sodium preferred also decreased ... these changes in taste occurred early and were evident by the sixth-week visit."

"In questionnaires, men on low-sodium diets reported they were more sensitive to the taste of salt, found many high salt foods to be unpleasant, and stated that the diet was easier to follow the longer they stayed on it," Grimm explained.

This confirms other studies that suggest our craving for salt is a learned behavior — an acquired taste. According to *High Blood Pressure Lowered Naturally* (FC&A Publishing), other studies with twins also show that salt craving is created by a high-salt diet.

It will take up to three months to completely lose the craving for salt, according to Mrs. Dash, a manufacturer of no-salt products.

The average American eats five to 10 grams of sodium, or one-third to one-fifth of an ounce of salt per day. This is much more salt than is needed for bodily functions. Most people only need one-tenth that amount. Many scientific studies show that reducing salt intake, ideally to 500 milligrams per day, will lower blood pressure in most people.

Processed foods, anything that comes in a can, a frozen package or a box, is likely to have salt added as a preservative or flavor enhancer.

---

## Tips to provide flavor without salt

- Use lemon juice on food instead of salt
- Use one of several salt-free mixtures of herbs and spices now available
- To spice chicken dishes, add fruit such as mandarin oranges or pineapples
- Marinate chicken, fish, beef or poultry in orange juice or lemon juice
- Use homemade mustard or honey to glaze meat dishes
- Use green pepper, parsley, paprika or red pepper
- In baking, use extracts instead of salt
- Learn about the many natural herbs, spices and fruit peels that are available

---

## Bran and other fiber lowers blood pressure

Daily fiber supplements helped lower high blood pressure, according to a recent study. Systolic pressure, the first number in blood pressure readings, dropped an average of 10 points, and the diastolic pressure, the second number, decreased an average of five points in just three months with fiber supplements, Danish researchers revealed in *Lancet* (2, 8559: 622). However, people in the control group of the study who took a placebo (a harmless, fake drug) experienced no change in their blood pressure levels.

Your fiber intake should be at least 30 grams each day and should include a variety of fiber types, according to the National Cancer Institute. Good sources of fiber include wheat bran, oat bran, fruits, vegetables (with skins), whole-grain breads, and cereals.

Until modern times, our ancestors ate a high-fiber diet, and many present-day digestive, colon, and bowel problems were rare in those days. Our digestive system is designed to handle a diet that contains bran, the outer fiber of cereal grains. Modern food processing methods remove much fiber from our food, which leads to constipation and other health problems, as well as high blood pressure.

Low-fiber diets have also been linked to heart and artery disease, constipation, appendicitis, colon cancer, diverticulosis, cancer of the large bowel, hemorrhoids, and obesity.

## Fish oil lowers 'mild' high blood pressure

High doses of fish oil lowered blood pressure in men with mild high blood pressure, according to a new study published in the *New England Journal of Medicine* (320,16:1037).

"We found that dietary supplementation with high doses of fish oil given for one month lowered blood pressure in men with mild essential hypertension, whereas a lower dose of fish oil, the same amount of safflower oil, or a mixture of saturated and unsaturated oils produced no significant change," reports Dr. Howard Knapp of Vanderbilt University.

The researchers compared the effect of the fish oil (15 grams daily, or slightly more than one-half ounce) with common prescription blood-pressure reducers. "The magnitude of the effect that we found was similar to that of propranolol or a thiazide diuretic in the Medical Research Council trial," Knapp says.

Although these results are promising, the researchers warn that "the clinical usefulness and safety of fish oil in the treatment of hypertension will require further study."

## Lowering high blood pressure: when can that be dangerous?

Just how much should high blood pressure be lowered? That's the question being asked by doctors at Albert Einstein College of Medicine in Bronx, N.Y. after a study there indicated some dangers associated with both big and small drops in blood pressure. The "moderate" declines seemed to be safest, says the report in the *Journal of the American Medical Association* (262,7:920).

Researchers say many more people eventually had severe or fatal heart attacks following blood pressure treatment that resulted in drops of less than six points or more than 18 points. Such people face three to four times the risk of heart attack, compared with those with moderate declines, the study says.

Seen in another way, the risks of fatal heart attack were

about the same for those whose high blood pressure remained virtually unchanged as for those with a large fall in blood pressure. Why those with big drops should face the same risks as those whose pressure remained high is unknown, the *JAMA* report says.

The research indicates that an "ideal" blood pressure figure may be an unrealistic goal and may even be dangerous for many people, according to a *New York Times* report of the study.

One speculation was that a big pressure drop may result in poor blood flow through heart arteries, starving the heart muscle and leading to a heart attack. They downplayed other possible factors like reaction to the medicines, other diseases and behavior like smoking and drinking. That's because those same factors were present in the ones who had moderate drops in pressure as well as in those who had small or large drops.

The doctors tracked 1,765 patients, three-quarters of them male and with an average age of 52 years. All patients had blood pressure higher than 160 systolic or 95 diastolic when they entered the study, the report says. Most of them took standard drug treatments, like diuretics, calcium channel blockers or beta blockers, to lower their blood pressure. But, "drug type mattered less than the magnitude of blood pressure decline," according to the *Times* report of the study.

The researchers say there was no direct time relationship between the big drop in blood pressure and a subsequent heart attack. Some attacks took place within a few weeks of the treatment; some occurred many months later.

The doctors make two suggestions:

(1) The attending doctor should seek a very specific treatment tailored to each patient that will protect the heart while trying to lower blood pressure, and

(2) "Until this goal is attainable, the cautious physician should seek modest (in the range of seven to 17 mm Hg of diastolic blood pressure) ... reduction for those with mild to moderate hypertension."

## Marriage helps protect against high blood pressure

Married people have an increased chance of surviving cancer.

Married couples also are less likely to have high blood pressure than people who are single, widowed, separated or divorced.

However, the researchers in several different studies are quick to say that they don't know exactly why marriage has such a positive effect on your health.

Unmarried people tend to wait longer to go to a doctor to be diagnosed, so their cancer is usually more advanced and more difficult to treat, doctors note. Unmarried people are also more likely than married people not to get any treatment at all, reports the *Journal of the American Medical Association* (258: 21, 3125).

Dr. James Goodwin, who has helped research several cancer studies, believes that marriage provides a support system and better finances for early diagnosis and treatment.

"It may simply be that married people live healthier lives," suggests Dr. Marjorie A. Speers. In a study by the Yale University Medical School and the University of Texas, where Speers is an assistant professor of preventative medicine, married people were 20 percent less likely to have high blood pressure than singles.

In the Speers study, married people were also more likely to know if they had high blood pressure, more likely to get treatment for it, and more likely to keep their high blood pressure under control.

It seems apparent that marriage is good for your health.

# Breathing and Lung Health

## Breathing fresh air may be harmful

Opening your windows for a breath of fresh air may be hazardous to your health. The fresher the air, the more it may harm you if you live in one of the 81 areas in the U.S. that flunk federal air-quality standards, according to reports in *Science News* (136,13:198) and *Medical World News* (30,18:39).

Bell Communications researchers in Red Bank, N.J., were baffled by laboratory equipment problems such as cracked power cords. Red Bank, incidentally, is just south of New York City, one of the nation's most polluted cities. To their surprise, the culprit was ozone, a type of oxygen.

To solve the mystery of the disintegrating equipment, Bell

researchers measured indoor ozone levels continuously, noting how many times per hour outdoor air was flushed through the company's buildings. Surprisingly, the "fresher" the air, the higher the ozone levels.

If you open the windows in your home, fresh air will be flushed through five times an hour, says Charles J. Weschler, a Bell senior scientist. People who spend a lot of time indoors and live in ozone-polluted areas may actually breathe more ozone indoors than out.

Inhaling ozone—whether indoors or out—for prolonged periods leads to lung inflammation and breathing problems. The effect of ozone and air pollution is like a sunburn, says Dr. Robert Phalen, who studies how dirty air affects health. Air pollution destroys the protective lining of the respiratory tract, from the nose down to the lungs, allowing poisons to enter the body more easily. After a lot of ozone exposure, the lungs "become far more susceptible to infection and cancer," says Dr. Phalen.

Other health problems include coughing, headache, eye irritation, sore throat and chest discomfort. The effects of pollution may be cumulative, meaning that illness may develop after years of exposure.

Ironically, people with healthy lungs may be more sensitive to ozone pollution than asthmatics, whose lungs are protected by a mucous lining. Also, people who exercise or do strenuous work in well-ventilated buildings may be more at risk because strenuous exercise causes heavy breathing and inhalation of unfiltered air through the mouth. (The nasal passages serve to filter air taken in through the nose.)

Air pollution, once thought to be an urban problem, affects

people living 100 miles downwind of a pollution source. The pollutants include ozone, sulfur dioxide and carbon monoxide. Weather patterns significantly affect air pollution across the U.S. Generally, winds blow west to east, resulting in more pollution in the east, according to the *Medical World News* report.

Doctors report that the number of asthma cases in the U.S. increased during the 1980s because of air pollution.

## Tips to protect yourself from ozone and air pollution

- Find out the daily pollution levels in your area from local newspapers, radio and TV stations. Call the National Weather Service Office or the nearest office of the Environmental Protection Agency to get more information on local pollution levels.
- If pollution levels are high, limit your time outdoors. Keep doors and windows closed during times of high levels of pollution.
- Consider installing air cleaning devices in your home, especially the devices that use activated charcoal to filter incoming air. Activated charcoal is a very good absorber for ozone. Don't confuse activated charcoal air cleaners with so-called "air purifiers." Most air purifiers don't trap ozone, radioactive radon gas or many of the other gases that cause health problems. Such devices do screen out larger airborne dust and pollen particles, but only

while the particles are in the air, not after they've settled on furniture and carpets.

- Don't use ozone-producing devices inside your home. Some ozone-producing devices are marketed as "air fresheners." They just add to the ozone pollution problem. Avoid them.
- Check with your doctor or health care provider about other options to protect your lungs if you have asthma or other breathing difficulties.

## Caution: some humidified air pollutes home

If you have one of the newer "high-tech" types of home humidifiers, here's a caution.

Fill your ultrasonic-wave humidifier with distilled or demineralized water, not water straight from your home faucet, according to a U.S. government scientist. If you use tap water in an ultrasonic humidifier, you could be polluting your indoor air with tiny mineral particles, says a report in *Science News* (134:141).

In a test conducted by researchers at the Environmental Protection Agency, an ultrasonic device filled with ordinary tap water sprayed an average room with 40 times the recommended safe limit for breathable mineral particles, the report says. Those mineral particles may include lead, aluminum and asbestos, all harmful if inhaled in high concentrations, the report says.

Traditional kinds of humidifiers, which use impellers or fan blades to break up moisture into fine particles, produce about one-third that amount, the report says. Steam vaporizer units didn't generate any measurable particles.

Using the ultrasonic humidifiers with regular tap water to help people with asthma may backfire and actually do more harm than good, say the researchers. Most makers of humidifiers advise using distilled or demineralized water, but many homeowners seem to be ignoring those warnings, the report says.

## The dirtiest areas in the U.S.

The Environmental Protection Agency recently released air pollution ratings for major U.S. cities, according to a report in *Medical World News* (30,18:42).

- **Severe pollution:** Chicago, Houston/Galveston, Los Angeles/Anaheim, New York City/Long Island/Northern N.J.

- **Serious pollution:** Atlanta; Baton Rouge; Boston; Cincinnati; El Paso; Louisville; Milwaukee; Portland; San Diego; Springfield, Mass.; Washington, D.C.

- **Moderate pollution:** Atlantic City; Birmingham, Ala.; Cleveland/Akron; Detroit; Grand Rapids, Michigan; Knoxville; Memphis, Tenn.; Miami; Phoenix; Raleigh/Durham, N.C.; Richmond; San Francisco

# Cigarette smoking increases stroke risk

Cigarette smokers have a three to four times greater risk of stroke than nonsmokers, Australian researchers report in *The Lancet* (2,8664:643). If you smoke two packs a day, your risk of stroke is twice that of someone the same age who smokes one pack a day; if you live with a smoker, you inhale passive smoke and also are at risk for stroke, researchers said. (This new information on health risks from passive smoking will no doubt heat up the smoking-in-public debate.)

Stroke occurs when blood flow to the brain is blocked, resulting in a loss of brain function. Stroke can cause paralysis, brain damage or death.

There are different types of stroke. Stroke may be caused by bleeding in the brain itself (a cerebral hemorrhage) or a blood clot that travels from the heart to the brain (a cerebral embolism). Hardening of the arteries in the brain or neck may lead to blockage of major blood vessels supplying the brain. This type of stroke is called a cerebral thrombosis, a major cause of which is smoking.

Researchers examined the relationship between cigarette smoking and stroke. In previous studies, chronic smoking was shown to break down the inner lining of arteries, causing blood to thicken and slow down, but has not been "consistently implicated" as a stroke risk factor.

They studied 844 people — 422 patients suffering their first stroke and 422 residents of the same area who had never had a stroke. The average age of the participants was 65. In choosing stroke patients for the study, researchers used sophisticated scanning equipment to determine what type of stroke the patient suffered.

Researchers interviewed participants about their previous diet and exercise, medical history, alcohol consumption and smoking habits (what they smoked, how much and how long). Of the stroke patients, 32 percent were current smokers, 34 percent were ex-smokers, and 34 percent had never smoked. Of the subjects who had never had a stroke, 18 percent were current smokers, 32 percent were ex-smokers, and 49 percent had never smoked, researchers said.

"Smoking, hypertension [high blood pressure], and a history of [heart attack] were significant and independent risk factors, whereas alcohol consumption seemed to have a modest but significant protective effect," the report concluded. The risk was slightly higher for men than women.

The risk for smokers was about the same as their risk of heart attack. For those who quit, the risk was still strong after 10 years. Researchers said that some of the effects of smoking are reversible, but because the stroke risk persists for 10 years or more, they think that smoking has more lasting effects than once believed.

## You can stop smoking with this 13-step system!

Even if you're a "hard core" smoker — someone over age

55 who's smoked for more than 30 years — you *can* stop. All it takes is motivation and a system that replaces old habits with new ones, say researchers in *Senior Patient* (1,5:36). In this report, they detail a system to help older smokers kick the habit. The system works, the researchers report, and the rewards are great.

A number of studies have shown that older Americans who quit smoking are less likely to develop heart disease and less likely to die from it. The disease rates "are significantly lower for ex-smokers than for current smokers," researchers say. "And quitting benefits general health and vitality."

Here's a 13-step system that will allow you to take control of your smoking habit:

(1) "Set a target quitting date." Choose a day you think that stress will be minimal and you won't be around other smokers.

(2) Once you've set a target date, "keep a record of your smoking habits, including the times and the places." Keeping a diary will help you recognize how much you smoke and why you smoke. Did a confrontation with a co-worker, rush-hour traffic or an upsetting phone call make you reach for your cigarettes?

(3) Designate a "smoking place" in your home and at work. "Smoke *only* in those places." Choose a place that is inconvenient and uncomfortable. One person chose the corner of his basement; another chose the front lawn. If it's raining or very cold, you might decide to stay indoors rather than smoke. And you will look silly standing there smoking on your front lawn.

(4) Keep ashtrays and lighters only in this designated smoking place.

(5) Don't carry cigarettes with you. Ask nonsmokers (spouse, co-workers) to hold your cigarettes. You will have to ask for a cigarette whenever you want one.

(6) Smoke alone and do nothing else (no watching television, drinking coffee or talking on the phone) while smoking. Take the pleasure out of the habit. Make smoking a chore.

(7) Change smoking postures. If you hold your cigarette in your right hand, switch to your left. If you draw from your cigarette on the left side of your mouth, switch to your right. These changes should make smoking more awkward and uncomfortable for you.

(8) "Buy one pack at a time," and buy lower-tar brands.

(9) "Delay your first smoke of the day and the first one after a meal. Start with a half-hour delay and work up to an hour."

(10) When you want a cigarette, "put off lighting it for a while. Hold it in your hand and tell yourself, 'I don't need to light this just yet.'" Once you begin to take control of your habit, the urge for a cigarette might pass.

(11) Set up a support network. Choose sympathetic friends (perhaps ex-smokers) whom you can call when you feel the urge for a cigarette.

(12) Start an exercise program to help prevent weight gain. But remember: Quitting is the goal. You can worry about any extra pounds later.

(13) "Reward yourself often" for accomplishing your goals.

If you cut down smoking before your target date arrives, quitting should be less stressful for you. If you have cold feet about this, talk to your doctor about prescribing nicotine gum, which will help control the urge to smoke.

Experts stress that you should use nicotine gum to quit smoking — not to cut down — because inhaled nicotine is more potent than the nicotine in chewing gum, and the gum will not work for you.

Quitting smoking takes time, especially if you are a long-term smoker. If your habit gets the best of you the first time, try again — and again. Don't lose your motivation to quit smoking. Researcher David Dworkin offers these words of wisdom to everyone trying to quit: "No one ever died from quitting smoking."

## Secret revealed — an easier way to stop smoking

Recent research may help you kick the smoking habit with a lot less grief from something called the tobacco withdrawal syndrome. The secret is this — at the same time you're cutting down on smoking and nicotine, cut way back on caffeine, too, according to a report in the *British Medical Journal* (298,6680:1075).

Researchers in San Francisco discovered that when you stop smoking, the caffeine levels in your blood skyrocket.

Sometimes the caffeine levels in the blood of recent quitters were two-and-a-half times the smoking levels.

The non-smoker's body doesn't burn off caffeine nearly so quickly as that of a smoker, doctors think. In fact, they believe, smokers have to drink a lot more caffeine than non-smokers do to get the same effect. The researchers studied 95 people and found that caffeine levels stayed about the same for those who continued smoking. But, "plasma caffeine concentrations increase after people give up smoking and remain increased for at least six months," the report says.

Studies show that smokers trying to kick the nicotine habit tend to load up on coffee and caffeine-containing drinks and foods. In effect, they increase their caffeine intake to compensate for the loss of nicotine.

Three or four days after a smoker kicks the smoking habit, her body metabolism slows down its caffeine-burning rate. Thus, the new non-smoker gets a much bigger jolt from her customary amount of caffeine than before she quit smoking— the equivalent of suddenly drinking two times as much coffee.

That's the problem. "Assuming that consumption of caffeine is unchanged, high caffeine concentrations could contribute to the tobacco withdrawal syndrome," the *BMJ* report says. That's like adding a few boulders to an already heavy backpack.

So when you quit smoking, cut your daily caffeine consumption by at least half. If you were used to drinking two cups of caffeinated coffee in the morning while you smoked, cut back to less than one full cup as your body adjusts to non-smoking. Watch out for caffeine in cola drinks and chocolate, too.

Trying to quit smoking is tough enough. Don't add to your woes — or even sabotage your new-found freedom from smoking — by getting too much caffeine at the same time, the report urges.

## Indoor tobacco smoke exposure may triple women's cancer risks

Smoking is hazardous not only to the smoker. Just being in the same room with tobacco smoke may be dangerous to non-smokers, especially women, according to two recent scientific studies.

Non-smoking women who have been exposed to "sidestream" or "passive" tobacco smoke run increased risks of developing both cancer of the cervix and breast cancer, the studies suggest.

Sidestream smoke, passive smoking, and involuntary smoking are all terms that mean the same thing, according to the U.S. Government's Office on Smoking and Health. The terms refer to the tobacco smoke that is inhaled without choice by a nonsmoking person, particularly inside a closed area like an office building or house.

Researchers at the University of Utah found that women exposed to passive smoke for more than three hours a day were three times more likely to develop cancer of the cervix, the opening from the vagina to the womb. The greatest risk was to women whose husbands or other household members smoked a lot. The study also found that women over age 40 faced a higher risk of getting cervical cancer from passive smoke than did women under 40.

The Utah study—reported in the *Journal of the American Medical Association* (261,11:1593)—ran for three years and involved 270 white women ages 20 through 59, all of whom had developed cancer of the cervix. The researchers compared the cancer patients' smoking exposure to that of a control group of 408 women without cancer.

Although the report in *JAMA* was careful not to blame smoking as the cause of cervical cancer, it did suggest that smoking may play a major role in the disease's development. The Utah study is the first to directly link passive smoking with cancer of the cervix, although some scientists have speculated about it for a decade. Passive smoke has already been linked to lung cancer.

A second statistical study says indoor tobacco smoke is a major risk factor in developing breast cancer. Although the female hormone estrogen is believed to play perhaps the leading role in breast cancers, passive smoking might be as high as second on the list, according to researcher A. Wesley Horton.

"Estrogen may be the principal promoter of human breast cancer," says Horton in a report in *Cancer* (62:6), "but evidence is mounting that indoor tobacco smoke can play a critical role." One out of every 10 American women will develop breast cancer, Horton reports.

Breast cancer is the second leading cause of death among women in the United States. Three out of every four breast cancer patients are over age 50. That puts a high priority on learning the causes of breast cancer and learning how to minimize the risk factors.

Horton, a professor at Oregon Health Sciences University, found that countries with high rates of lung cancer in men also have high rates of breast cancer in women, even when the women were not smokers. Countries with low rates of lung cancer in men also had low rates of breast cancer in women.

Although women can be exposed to sidestream smoke at home or at work, smoke from their husbands' cigarettes was the largest factor in breast cancer patients, Horton reports. "The increased cancer risk from the passive inhalation of sidestream smoke is not limited to nonsmokers, but is significantly increased in smokers, too," a fact Horton attributes to D.P. Sandler in the *American Journal of Epidemiology* (121:37 and 123:370).

Horton believes that inhaling passive smoke may be more dangerous than actually smoking a cigarette. "Some of the chemical initiators (that cause cancer) are much more concentrated in sidestream than in mainstream tobacco smoke," Horton says. Mainstream smoke is that smoke inhaled directly by the smoker.

Horton's report says it usually takes more than 20 years of inhaling passive tobacco smoke before a nonsmoking woman develops breast cancer. According to that report, the current rates of breast cancer could have been influenced by indoor, passive smoke inhalation during the late 1960s and early 1970s.

Horton's study offers comfort to women "whose parents, housemates, and employers provided them smoke-free households and workplaces." Furthermore, he suggests that "those who remained nonsmokers probably have a much lower risk of breast cancer than the one in 10 cited previously."

As for smokers, Horton urges them to "practice" their habit outdoors. "Designated smoking areas" and air-conditioning with "recirculation of smoke-contaminated air more than doubles ... exposure to sidestream smoke," he concludes.

## Baking soda and water may help you kick the smoking habit

One of the biggest barriers to people trying to stop smoking is the physical discomfort of nicotine withdrawal.

Those discomforts include headaches, nervous "jitters," an actual craving for a nicotine "kick" and increased irritability, among other things.

Withdrawal can be eased by a prescription drug called Nicorette. Usually found in the form of chewing gum, Nicorette slowly releases a measured dose of nicotine into the body to cut the craving for nicotine from a smoke.

Ask your doctor if this prescription drug would be safe and appropriate for you.

Another way to ease off the nicotine habit is to take a half teaspoonful of bicarbonate of soda in a glass of water two or three times a day.

Apparently, the bicarbonate of soda mixed in water helps to hold nicotine in the system and reduce withdrawal symptoms by giving the body more time to adapt to doing without nicotine.

Once a smoker has successfully withdrawn from tobacco for two weeks, most withdrawal symptoms should pass.

Be sure to check with your doctor and get his approval before trying this method.

A reminder: cut back on caffeine-containing drinks and foods while you are trying to kick the smoking and nicotine habit.

Clinical tests indicate that caffeine in your system might worsen your nicotine withdrawal symptoms and just add to your cravings for a cigarette.

Regular aerobic exercise, such as running, walking, playing tennis, swimming, bike riding and hard physical labor, can help you kick the smoking habit.

Begin to associate with non-smokers as an aid in maintaining your determination to quit smoking and in resisting all temptations to start puffing again.

As well as reducing your risks of long-term health problems, there are immediate benefits to quitting smoking.

You will be able to breathe more easily, and you'll find you have greater endurance when participating in sports or exercise.

Your senses of taste and smell improve.

The stains on your hands and teeth disappear, and your breath gets sweeter.

After you quit, you will have fewer colds, and within two weeks you should notice an improvement in your "smoker's hack" or cough.

# Cancer, General

## Cancer prevention tips

- Avoid drinking or cooking with chlorinated water
- Avoid using talcum powder in the genital areas
- Avoid drinking coffee, either regular or decaffeinated
- Avoid contact with asbestos
- Avoid excessive exposure to the sun
- Avoid fried foods
- Avoid processed foods containing carcinogenic additives
- Avoid barrier forms of contraception
- Eat foods rich in vitamin D, calcium, molybdenum, and selenium, such as fish, whole grain foods, wheat germ, and beans
- Include lysine, an amino acid, in your diet
- Eat crunchy, yellow and dark-green leafy vegetables
- Reduce sodium and increase potassium in your diet
- Eat foods rich in dietary fiber

• Avoid cigarettes
• Avoid excessive amounts of alcohol

Source — *Natural Health and Wellness Encyclopedia*, FC&A Publishing, 1988.

# Preventing cancer: your diet can make the difference

Despite ever-increasing evidence that what we eat can play a major role in preventing many forms of cancer, only about one in five Americans regularly eats the right kinds of foods to get the highest protection.

Researchers at the National Cancer Institute in Bethesda, Md. surveyed 11,658 white and black adults about a typical day's diet. The study showed that only 16 percent of those surveyed ate high-fiber cereals or whole-grain breads. Only 18 percent ate at least one green vegetable (high in cancer-fighting beta carotene), and only 20 percent had any kind of fibrous vegetables. High vitamin C fruits and vegetables came out a little better (28 percent).

On the other hand, 55 percent of all adults ate red meat, rich in cholesterol, at least once a day. Processed lunch meats and breakfast, both high in many suspected cancer-causing preservatives, appeared on the menus of 49 percent of the males and 37 percent of the females surveyed.

The large study showed, in fact, that many of us tend to eat just those things that are worst for our health and avoid those foods that are best for us.

Income levels and where we live make a difference, the study showed. Southerners balanced a plus with a minus, eating the least red meat but ignoring high-fiber cereals. Young white males seem to avoid foods that are good sources of vitamins A and C. The higher the income, the more red meat, produce and high-fiber cereals are consumed.

Numerous scientific studies advise us to eat fruits and vegetables, whole grains and foods rich in vitamins A and C and fiber, and to do it every day. The same studies say we should cut way down on red meats and fat and avoid any foods that have been salt-cured, nitrite-cured, smoked or pickled.

On the same lines, a report in the *American Journal of Clinical Nutrition* (49,5:993) outlines how your diet can mean the difference between healthy maturity and lingering illnesses.

About 35 percent of all cancers currently are linked to poor diet, according to the report. A high-fiber diet has been shown to reduce colon-cancer risk, and a high-fat diet increases breast-cancer risk. The experts have devised "interim" dietary guidelines, which include a varied, well-balanced diet (fruits, vegetables, whole grains) with reduced fat, salt, alcohol and processed foods.

You should also watch your weight.

## Cabbages, collards and cancer

Several studies have shown that some common vegetables like cabbages and collards fight the formation of cancerous tumors. In particular, big cabbage eaters have higher than normal protection against cancers of the stomach, breast and colon. Animal studies showed increased protection against cancer of the lung for animals fed diets rich in cabbage and cauliflower.

Now, a new study in the journal *Nutrition and Cancer* (12,2:121) demonstrates that a diet including cabbage and collards protects against the spread of breast cancer to the lungs. This study, involving rats, is the first to show that a diet that includes a particular family of vegetables fights the spread of cancer cells from its original location to another site in the body.

"The metastasis, or spread of a tumor to a secondary site, is the cause of death of a majority of patients, despite removal or treatment of the primary tumor with chemotherapy or radiation," the report says.

All the animals got injections of live breast cancer cells. Then the researchers watched to see how many in each group would develop cancer of the lungs as a result of the spread of the cancer cells. At the end of the two-month experiment, animals fed cabbages and collards had half as many lung tumors as the rats fed a control diet without the two vegetables. The researchers said they felt collards and cabbage diets might be useful in treating active cancerous tumors in addition to fighting the spread of the disease.

Cabbages and collards are both in a family known as cruciferous vegetables. Cruciferous vegetables get their name from the scientific term for plants whose flowers have petals in the shape of a cross. Cruciferae is the Latin name meaning "cross-bearing."

Among the many edible plants in this family are cabbage, cauliflower, collards, broccoli, Brussels sprouts, kohlrabi, kale and radish.

## Onions and garlic may be
## natural cancer fighters

You may not like what onions and garlic do to your breath. But your stomach and colon may be dying for what these members of the allium family can contribute to better health.

Scientists at the National Cancer Institute, working with colleagues in China, discovered that Chinese who eat a lot of onions and garlic have only a fourth as many stomach cancers as other Chinese. That's important, because the Chinese population has a high rate of stomach cancers, according to a report of the findings in *Healthline* (8,8:5).

Researchers are still trying to determine what it is about onions, garlic, chives, leeks and scallions that seems to slash the numbers of such deadly cancers. One NCI official suspects that the protective agent is the smelly part of the vegetables, the allyl sulfides, according to another report in *Health* (21,5:16).

Scientists at the University of California, Berkeley, think the answer may lie with a turncoat chemical, quercetin. Quercetin switches sides in the cancer battle, sometimes acting like a powerful cancer causer, other times like a strong cancer fighter. It's found in alliums and in deep green and yellow vegetables like broccoli and squash. It also turns up in red grapes and in common plants like ferns. Onions are extremely high in the substance.

In ferns and red wine (made from fermented grapes), quercetin seems to be a mutagen, a chemical that helps to trigger cancerous tumors. In fruits and vegetables, quercetin ties in with natural sugars and takes on a neutral stance, neither causing nor fighting cancer.

But once those sugar-linked quercetin molecules get into the digestive system, our natural enzymes break down the sugars and release quercetin into the stomach and intestines. Some bacterial enzymes present in our digestive tract act differently or not at all with different foods. For example, some bacteria work only with milk products. What quercetin does to our insides — whether it acts as friend or foe — may depend on what kinds of natural bacteria we have inside us and on what combinations of food we eat, the Berkeley scientists think.

Apparently, the alliums and quercetin act as allies against cancer. But researchers say more study is needed to see what exactly goes on. Meanwhile, consider adding more onions and garlic to your recipes, says the *Health* story.

## Milk sugar can be a cancer risk

Women who have trouble digesting a form of sugar found in dairy products may face higher risks of developing cancer of the ovaries, a study in *Lancet* ((2,8654:66) suggests. The study is the first to link dairy products to ovarian cancer, says

*Science News* (136,4:52).

The researchers "found that women who ate yogurt at least once a month were nearly twice as likely to develop ovarian cancer as women who reported less frequent yogurt consumption," according to the *SN* report. Eating cottage cheese at least once a month also raised the cancer risk, the report says. The culprit may be galactose, a type of dairy sugar, the researchers say.

Some women have trouble producing a digestive enzyme to break down the galactose, according to the study. Many don't even know they have the problem.

But if they eat dairy products, this disability may result in "potentially toxic galactose bathing their ovaries for longer than women who metabolize the sugar efficiently," says the *SN* report. "Women who consumed more dairy products than they could metabolize had the greatest risk of ovarian cancer," the report says.

People get the bulk of galactose during digestion of lactose, the main sugar found in milk products. A little galactose is found naturally in most dairy products.

But yogurt and cottage cheese contain higher amounts of galactose. That's because a natural bacteria process breaks down the lactose and releases galactose during the making of the two products.

If the surprising findings are backed up by other studies, "avoidance of lactose-rich foods by adults may be a way of primary prevention of ovarian cancer," says Harvard Medical School researcher Dr. Daniel W. Cramer, one of the authors of the study.

# Study links bone cancer to fluoride

Flying in the face of 50 years of government and scientific acceptance, a new federally-sponsored study suggests that fluoride may have caused bone cancers in some laboratory test animals, reports *Medical Tribune* (30,31:1).

"Very preliminary data from recent health studies on fluoride indicate that fluoride may be a carcinogen," the *Tribune* quotes from a briefing paper prepared by staff scientists at the Environmental Protection Agency. A carcinogen is a chemical that harms body tissue and triggers cancer.

"If fluoride turns out to be a carcinogen, it will be the environmental story of the century," the story quotes an official of the American Water Works Association. The AWWA is a group that represents the nation's municipal and public water suppliers.

The EPA just last year raised the allowable limit of fluoride in public water supplies.

More than six out of every 10 public water suppliers routinely add fluoride to drinking water in a campaign to cut tooth decay. Many of them have been fluoridating water since the 1940s, the *Tribune* report says.

In addition, most toothpastes contain added fluorides, and dentists across the country routinely prescribe fluoride supplements for pregnant women and many children, the paper says.

The fluoridation campaign, despite outcries from various

groups in the '40s and '50s, has gained wide medical and public acceptance.

In recent months, the EPA has come under criticism for seeming to ignore some studies that showed disturbing links between fluoridated water and increased cancer rates, the news report says.

For example, in the late '70s, a scientific study showed that cities with fluoridated water supplies had a 5 percent increase in cancer rates. Other studies have been less clear.

Meanwhile, the EPA is planning a full review of its fluoride standards during 1990, and may tighten its liberal 1986 limits on fluoride levels in drinking water, the report says.

Fluoride is a compound made from the gaseous element fluorine. It's a chemical cousin to chlorine, which is used in most public water supplies to kill bacteria in drinking water.

Fluoride gets into and chemically bonds with teeth and bones. It seems to strengthen teeth and make them less vulnerable to decay.

Its reputation for fighting tooth decay has been the main justification for adding the chemical to more than half the nation's water supplies.

So far the strongest evidence linking fluoride to bone cancer comes strictly from animal tests.

However, the government banned some artificial sweeteners during the past two decades based strictly on animal tests that showed links to cancer.

# New study tells more about cigarettes and cancer

It's been suspected for years that it's the high-tar, high-nicotine content in cigarette smoke that causes most of the damage to smokers' lungs. A new study in *Preventive Medicine* (18,4:518) adds new weight to that belief.

"Tar (is) the main carcinogenic agent in cigarette smoke," the researchers say. They further charge that lung cancer risk rises in a direct line with tar content in cigarette smoke. In other words, the higher the tar level of the cigarette, the greater the risk of getting lung cancer.

Most American smokers have switched to so-called low-tar brands in recent years, the study says. Most low-tar brands are filter-tipped. One estimate says that the average male smoker inhales a filtered smoke containing 13.8 milligrams of tar. The average woman smoker puffs a cigarette that delivers to her lungs 11.8 milligrams of tar. At that level of tar intake, a 10-cigarette-a-day smoker would be about five times more likely to develop deadly lung cancer than a non-smoker, according to a risk chart in the new study.

Cigarette smoking is blamed for 85 percent of lung cancer cases in men and for 75 percent of such cases in women, according to the American Cancer Society. Besides lung cancer, the number one cancer killer, smoking has been strongly linked to cancers of the larynx (the voice box), esophagus and bladder.

"Smoking accounts for about 30 percent of all cancer deaths," says *Postgraduate Medicine* (86,2:213). Smokers who puff two or more packs a day die from lung cancer 15 to 25 times more often than non-smokers, according to the journal report.

Smoking has been called the number one reversible cause of death in the world.

## B vitamins may offer protection from cancer

The B family of vitamins may fight tumor formation and boost protection from cancer, according to a nutrition scientist. That's important "because 30 to 40 percent of cancers in men and up to 60 percent of cancers in women are related in some way to diet," *Food and Nutrition News* (61,3:15) reports.

"The B-complex vitamins appear to have supportive roles in maintaining immune system functions which can aid in preventing growth of initiated tumors, as well as having anticancer effects of their own," researcher Ronald Ross Watson writes in *Food and Nutrition News*.

"A balanced diet consisting of moderate amounts of a wide variety of wholesome foods, including those containing the B-complex vitamins ... will enhance health and offer protection against the devastating disease of cancer," Watson says.

• **Pyridoxine (vitamin B6)** — "Of all the B-complex vitamins, vitamin B6 appears to have the most important role in maintaining the normal functioning of the immune system," says Watson. Deficiencies of vitamin B6 possibly decrease resistance to cancer and other diseases. In addition, vitamin B6 is being tested as a treatment for melanoma skin cancer.

- **Folic acid** — Increased intake of folic acid might decrease the occurrence of cancer, some researchers believe.

That's because people with folic acid deficiencies have higher rates of stomach cancer and cancer of the esophagus, the tube from the mouth to the stomach.

Folic acid supplements have also been used to successfully treat cervical dysplasia, a precancerous condition of the opening to the womb, according to *Food and Nutrition News*.

- **Vitamin B12** — "A recent preliminary study in smokers who had potentially precancerous lung lesions implicated a role for folic acid and vitamin B12 in (lowering) the risk of lung cancer," Watson says. "Vitamin B12 is also thought to support immune system functions", he says, but its unique role is difficult to identify because vitamin B12 works and interacts so closely with folic acid.

- **Thiamine (Vitamin B1)** — "Animal experiments have shown that a deficiency of thiamine may cause immune system impairment," and could play a possible role in the development of human cancer, the study reveals.

- **Riboflavin (Vitamin B2)** — "Certain populations of people in China, Africa and Iran who have dietary deficiencies of vitamin B2 have shown a high incidence of esophageal cancer," according to Watson. Riboflavin is important in the development and maintenance of certain cells in the esophagus. In some cases, riboflavin supplements helped shrink cancer sores, but more research is needed in this area, he says.

"Whole grains, nuts, beans, lean meats, milk, eggs and leafy green vegetables are good sources of B vitamins," according to the article.

"The risk of cancer may be expected to be increased if people avoid certain healthful foods, such as dairy products, lean meats and nuts," just because these foods are high in calories or fat, Watson warns. In any diet you follow, make sure you get the recommended daily minimums of essential vitamins and minerals.

## Vitamins that may fight cervical cancer

Women with abnormal cervical cells sometimes have low blood levels of vitamin A, vitamin C, and folic acid, one of the B vitamins. These abnormal cells, known as cervical dysplasia, can develop into cancer of the cervix in women. The cervix is the opening to the womb.

Research is now underway at Albert Einstein College of Medicine in New York to see if adding these vitamins to the diet can help reverse the abnormal cell development and help prevent cervical cancer.

Other studies have linked low levels of vitamin A to development of cervical cancer, according to reports in *Gynecology and Oncology* (30,2:187) and *American Journal of*

*Obstetrics and Gynecology* (148,3:309). But this new research will focus on the role of vitamin supplements in preventing cervical cancer.

## Too much iron may cause cancer

Iron supplements should be avoided unless people have a deficiency, new research suggests. A recent report says unusually high doses of iron have been linked to greater human cancer risks.

A report in the *New England Journal of Medicine* (319:1047) warns that excess amounts of iron stored in the body may cause an increased risk of cancer and death, particularly in men. In a study involving 14,000 people over 13 years, the researchers linked high body levels of iron with cancer of the colon, bladder, esophagus and lungs.

Unlike most other vitamins and minerals, iron is not automatically thrown off by the body, but is stored. Therefore, taking too much iron can cause unhealthy iron deposits in the body.

People with low levels of iron in their blood, known as anemia, often take several iron supplements daily. Supplements also are recommended after surgery, blood loss, for people with hemorrhoids, peptic ulcers, or colitis, or for women with heavy menstrual periods. The U.S. Government also recommends extra iron for women during pregnancy and breast feeding. Additional iron is very important for the health of these people.

However, other people take iron as part of their daily vitamin and mineral intake, or just because they feel that more iron will help keep them healthy. But iron supplements for people who are not anemic may be unwise, Dr. Richard G. Stevens, stated in the journal.

Many foods, like breakfast cereals, often have added iron. Because of the possible link with cancer, Stevens questioned whether everyday foods should be "iron fortified."

## Nasal sprays and cancer

People using nose sprays were nearly four times more likely to develop cancers of the nasal passages and sinus areas than non-users, according to a study reported in the *Journal of Epidemiology and Community Health* (42:243).

The study showed that cancer risk rose as nose spray usage increased. The longer people used the preparations, and the more weeks out of the year that they sprayed themselves, the greater the risk of developing cancer, the report said.

People who had been using sprays or drops for 10 years faced a risk six times greater than those who had used sprays or drops less than one year. Those who used sprays or drops up to 26 weeks each year had a risk factor 3.8 times greater than those who used the preparations less than one week a year.

Many of those studied used the nose drops and sprays to fight nasal congestion and runny noses brought on by hay fever and colds. The preparations included decongestants and corticosteroids, and contained a mixture of over-the-counter medicines and prescription drugs.

The researchers said most of the cancer tumors were squamous cell type, the kind that develop in the surface layer of tissues lining the nasal and sinus passages. They compared a group of 53 people with sinonasal cancers with a larger group of 552 people without cancer who had no history of nasal medication use. The study was done in western Washington state.

Another study reported in *Healthline* (7,4:14) found that over-the-counter nose sprays can be addictive. A doctor at Stanford University Medical Center Allergy Clinic says that prolonged use of decongestants causes nose tissues to swell up even after both the spray and the condition that caused the nose irritation are removed. This "rebound" effect makes a person's nose feel stuffed up even when the cold or flu has long gone, the study said.

The clinic's advice: don't use nose sprays for more than three days.

## Where you live can prevent cancer

Where you live can help prevent cancer or can increase your risk of developing cancer. If you live in the northeastern United States, you are at higher risk of developing breast and colon cancer than Southerners or Westerners, according to research from the American Cancer Society.

Benzopyrine, a pollutant generated by automotive exhaust, tobacco smoke, and power and industrial plants, has been identified as starting and promoting cancer development, according to a study by biochemist Jack Bartley in Berkeley, Calif. It is found in higher concentrations in the Northeast.

Even if you don't live in an area with air pollution, where you live can still be dangerous. Radon gas in homes may be the second leading cause of lung cancer, according to the Environmental Protection Agency (EPA).

Radon gas is a radioactive by-product of uranium and radium that has been found in over 30 states. It is a colorless, odorless gas that can seep undetected into a house through concrete floors, floor drains, cracks, or even through your water, if you have a private well. Radon is absorbed into your lungs by breathing contaminated smoke and dust particles.

To check your home's radon gas level, call your local health department or the Radon Information Service sponsored by the EPA at 1-800-334-8571 (ext. 7131). Some "do-it-yourself" radon testing kits are now available on the market so you can test your own home for contamination.

Also check your neighborhood for large chemical plants, polluted water, or waste disposal areas. Living close to these places increases your risk of getting cancer.

## Common U.S. fern linked to high cancer rates

The bracken fern, one of the world's most common plants,

has been linked to cancer in animals who eat it and to high rates of cancer in people who live or work in bracken-covered areas, the *Medical Tribune* (30,6:2) reports.

Two field guides to edible wild plants in America recommend eating this plant, either cooked or raw. A recent report from Europe, however, accuses the same plant of being a potent cancer-causer. "Deer, cattle and sheep that graze on bracken develop mouth and stomach cancers," the article says.

Studies from Costa Rica and Venezuela showed that people who drink milk from cows that have grazed on bracken, in turn, develop more cancers of the stomach and esophagus, the *Tribune* article says.

The fern under fire is known scientifically as Pteridium aquilinum and is commonly known in this country as pasture brake, eagle fern, brakes, hog brake and brake fern. It is the single most common wild fern in the United States.

It grows easily in "full sunlight, in woods, old pastures, new roadsides, burned-over regions, sandy and partially shaded areas and in thickets," according to *Field Guide to Edible Wild Plants* (Stackpole Books, 1974: pg. 158), a manual still being sold in many bookstores.

Still another manual, *Field Guide to North American Edible Wild Plants* (Outdoor Life Books, 1982: pg. 58) lists bracken as a "related edible species" to ostrich fern. In that guide, bracken was considered a non-poisonous plant.

Even getting close to bracken may be hazardous, the *Tribune* report suggests. One expert recommends that anyone who goes often into areas in which bracken covers the ground should wear a face mask to limit exposure to bracken spores.

The spores are thought to contain several powerful cancer-causing substances such as shikimik milk, quercetin and ptaquiloside.

That face mask group should include "shepherds, forestry workers, and even hikers and backpackers," according to Dr. Jim Taylor of University College in Wales (Great Britain) and chairperson of the International Bracken Group.

"People may also be affected by drinking water from bracken-covered slopes" and by drinking milk from cows who have eaten bracken, he warns.

Bracken is one of the first ferns to appear in the spring. It grows to a height of from one to four feet, adding new leaves throughout the warm months. The darkly green fronds look heavy and leathery.

The fern spreads by oozing a toxic chemical into the ground that poisons all surrounding plants competing for the same space. These same poisons can affect both animals and people, according to the *Tribune* report.

The potentially dangerous spores are released from the maturing plant from June through October, Taylor says.

A further note — much research has been done on cancer-causing chemicals in recent years. Anyone who relies on field guides for safely stalking wild asparagus and other such wild delicacies should be sure the material has been printed very recently and contains the most up-to-date scientific information.

Check with your doctor or an expert in plant-produced chemicals about questionable plants. Safest bet of all — if it's wild, don't eat it. And, in the case of bracken fern, don't even get near it.

# Your job may increase your risk of bladder cancer

Painters, auto workers and drill press operators are just a few of the workers with an increased bladder-cancer risk, according to a new study in the *Journal of the National Cancer Institute* (81,19:1472).

Bladder cancer is the fifth deadliest cancer among men in the U.S. It's four times more common in men than in women.

Researchers at the National Cancer Institute in Bethesda, Md., interviewed 2,100 white men and 126 nonwhite men with bladder cancer to determine the type of jobs they had held for six months or more since age 12. They then compared that information with questionnaires completed by healthy men of the same age and race.

Among white men, high-risk occupations include driving trucks and taxicabs; grading and packing produce; performing railroad, lumberyard and insulation work; and broadcasting.

Among nonwhite men, auto workers, dry cleaners and clerical workers were at highest risk. The risk to petroleum workers was high in both groups.

Although researchers admit the relationship between job and bladder cancer may be coincidental in some cases, they estimate that "21–25 percent of bladder cancer diagnosed among white men in the United States is attributable to occupational exposures." For nonwhite men, that estimate jumps to 27 percent.

"Overall, our findings suggest that occupational bladder cancer among white and nonwhite men is similar," researchers say.

Smoking among all high-risk workers increased the cancer risk even more, they add.

The high-risk occupations have one thing in common: they expose workers to cancer-causing agents, such as dyes, air pollutants and toxic fumes. For example, painters are exposed to formaldehyde and asbestos, bootblacks to dyes in shoe polish, truck drivers to motor exhaust, machinery operators to coolants and lubricants used in cutting metal, and dry cleaners to petroleum-based cleaning solvents. Asbestos may contribute to insulation workers' increased risk.

Researchers failed to explain why the risk was high for workers such as clerks and broadcasters.

Among occupations studied, the length of time employed was significant in 16 categories. The odds of developing bladder cancer were greater for painters who began work before 1930 and who worked for more than 10 years. The same held true for petroleum processors.

# Breast Cancer

## High risk factors for breast cancer

Dense breast tissue increases the risk of breast cancer about fourfold, according to new research from the Centers for Disease Control (CDC) in Atlanta. "Women whose mammograms showed over 65 percent dense tissue developed breast cancer at a rate more than 400 percent higher than women with densities of less than 5 percent," Audrey F. Saftlas of the CDC and John N. Wolfe at the Hutzel Hospital in Detroit report in *Science News* (135,14:213).

If mammograms can be used to identify dense tissue and alert women with such dense tissue about their increased risks of breast cancer, this discovery can be very useful in helping to prevent this cancer, according to *Science News* .

Dense breast tissue "is at least as important as family

history" in determining a woman's risk for breast cancer, Saftlas says. Women with a family history of breast cancer are at highest risk, according to the *Journal of the American Medical Association* (253:1908).

In addition to having dense breast tissue, if you fall into one of the other high-risk categories listed below, be sure to get regular mammograms:

- If you gave birth to your first child after the age of 30.
- If you never gave birth.
- If your mother or sister has developed breast cancer.
- If you reached sexual maturity very early.
- If you have a history of cysts in your breasts.
- If you are overweight.
- If you are over 40 years of age.

## How to detect breast cancer early

Early detection is very important in surviving breast cancer, especially if you are at high risk. Have regular mammograms and examine your breasts every month.

The American Cancer Society now recommends that women 50 and over should have a mammogram once every year. Women between 40 and 49 should have a mammogram every second year. The first mammogram should be given when a woman is between 35 and 39 years of age. This will be used as a baseline to detect any irregularities later, the Cancer Society explains. A mammogram is a special x-ray of the breast which enables doctors to detect the earliest and most curable breast cancer.

Since a woman knows her own breasts, it is easier for her to detect changes in her breast tissue than for her doctor. Examining your breasts each month, in addition to your doctor's exam once a year, will help detect changes as early as possible. Besides lumps, watch for other possible signs of cancer including:

- Any change in the shape, size or color of the breasts. Do this by comparing them in a mirror each month. Compare them to each other and to how they looked the previous month.
- Any unusual discharge should be noted and reported to your doctor.
- Scaliness or crustiness on the breasts, especially around the nipple.
- Any new dimples in the breasts.
- Any lumps or thickening of the breast tissue.
- Asymmetry — any difference in the shapes of the breasts.

## A dietary secret that may prevent breast cancer

Can you change your diet and prevent breast cancer? Some researchers are saying cautiously that such a dietary prevention plan may be good ammunition against one of the biggest killers of women. The secret — lower the amount of fat you eat, suggest two studies.

"Dietary fat is a risk factor for breast cancer," conclude researchers in an Israeli study of 2,300 women. In general, the Israeli study shows that women with high-fat intakes are three times as likely to develop the types of tumors that turn into breast cancer. A high-fat diet promotes a change from benign (non-cancerous) breast disease to cancer, the researchers report in the *American Journal of Clinical Nutrition* (50,3:551). They point out that breast cancer develops in stages over a number of years, and if diet influences the process, women may be able to change their diet to help prevent cancer.

Diet apparently had no effect on two types of benign breast disease. But, among those with the most advanced stage (grade 3) of benign breast disease, they spotted a link between high-fat diets and numbers of women with breast cancer.

"The results suggest that saturated fatty acids, but not the other food groups, are associated with grade 3 disease," according to the report. Although women with grade 3 disease ate more starches, sugars and proteins than other women, their fat intake was the greatest risk factor, the researchers conclude.

In a separate study published in the *Journal of the National Cancer Institute* (81:278), Dr. Paolo Toniolo of the Department of Environmental Medicine at New York University Medical Center studied over 700 Italian women by analyzing their daily diet in 70 food categories.

Most strongly linked to increased rates of breast cancer were dairy products like high-fat cheese and whole milk, he reports. Ranked just under dairy products were fats and meat.

Women who ate foods rich in animal fat, such as meat and cured meat, showed a "modest" increase in the risk of breast cancer. "Consumption of fish, eggs, bread, pasta, olive oil, vegetables, and fruit did not reveal any evident relationship with breast cancer," the study says.

To reduce the risk of breast cancer, women need to reduce their consumption of total fat to less than 30 percent of their total daily calorie intake, saturated fat to less than 10 percent, and animal proteins to less than 6 percent, Toniolo suggests. The current typical American diet relies on fats for between 35 and 45 percent of total caloric intake.

Breast cancer develops from benign tumors. Although numerous studies have shown that a high-fat diet influences the process, researchers are not sure how. They do know that breast-cancer patients in Japan have better outcomes than their counterparts in the U.S. One possible reason for the difference is that Japanese women generally eat a relatively low-fat diet. Obesity and low-fiber, low-carbohydrate diets may also contribute to lower survival rates, researchers speculate.

A high-fat diet also may affect the recovery rates of women who undergo breast cancer surgery, according to a related study in the *Journal of the National Cancer Institute* (81,16:1218). Swedish researchers evaluated the diets of 240 women aged 50 to 65 who had breast-cancer surgery between 1983 and 1986, says the *JNCI* report. They were particularly interested in protein, carbohydrate, fat, alcohol and vitamin intake, but they also considered other factors such as height, weight, smoking and physical activity.

Women with larger tumors reported eating less fiber,

carbohydrates and vitamin A but more fat than women with smaller tumors. The high-fat eaters generally had larger tumors that spread farther, the research indicates. Women who drank alcohol also showed an increased risk, researchers said.

This is also affirmed in a report in *Science News* (134:100) that says eating a lot of saturated fats makes active breast cancer grow faster and spread farther, especially among older women. Canadian researchers studied the progress of recently diagnosed breast cancers in 666 women. Those with diets high in the kind of fats found in butter, cheese, and coconut oil developed larger cancers that spread more rapidly to the lymph nodes, indicating a more severe (and less curable) form of the disease. The more cancer involves the lymph nodes, the harder it is to get rid of the disease.

On the other hand, those who ate foods high in polyunsaturated fats — such as corn, safflower, sunflower, and cottonseed oils — showed less invasion of the lymph tissues, the report said, indicating a more treatable form of the disease.

On the positive and preventive side, another study reported in *Journal of the National Cancer Institute* (October 1988) showed that women who ate a "very low-fat diet" for a year developed fewer than half as many breast cancers as those who ate the "typical" diet. The low-fat diet apparently cut the cancer rate in half. Nearly 40 percent of the calories consumed in the "typical" American diet is in the form of fats, way too high for long-term health, the studies indicate.

According to the *JNCI* report, doctors at two Toronto hospitals put half of a group of 180 women whose mammograms showed unusual breast shadows on a specially formulated low-fat diet. Only about 20 percent of the diet's total calories was in the form of fat, while 56 percent was in carbohydrate form. The other half of the group, all of whom were diagnosed as facing higher risks of developing breast cancer, stuck to the "typical" diet — 37 percent of its calories in fat and 43 percent in carbohydrates.

After a year, five on the "typical" diet developed breast cancer, but only two on the low-fat diet came down with the disease, the Toronto study showed. A larger, follow-up study is planned.

While many studies have demonstrated higher risks of getting breast cancer because of fat-rich eating habits, the Canadian research is among the first to show that the growth and spread of the cancer is affected by what we eat — **after the cancer has become active.**

This suggests that a low-fat diet could be an important weapon in fighting breast cancer, even after it has been diagnosed. The studies also hint that a low-fat diet over many months (1) could lower the risk of getting breast cancer; (2) could lessen the severity of the disease once it's active; and (3) could even increase the cure rate.

## Vitamin D treatment may slow spread of breast cancer cells

Investigators in England saw good results when they treated breast cancer cells in the laboratory with vitamin D three times a week. More than 80 percent of all breast cancer tumors contain chemical "sockets" that plug in with the vitamin D, said the report in *The Lancet* (1, 8631:188).

Vitamin D in one form acts like a hormone in a woman's body, and attaches to hormonally-dependent tumors, they said. Once attached to a tumor, the vitamin D acts to halt spread of cancer cells and works to return cell activity to normal, the report said.

## Long-term estrogen therapy linked to breast cancer

Many menopausal women take estrogen to prevent osteoporosis and heart and circulatory problems, but Swedish researchers have found a link between the hormone and breast cancer, leaving women and their physicians to decide whether estrogen's benefits outweigh the risks, suggest reports in *New England Journal of Medicine* (321,5:293) and *Science* (245,4918:593).

Because American women generally take a different form of estrogen than do Swedish women, no one knows the impact of the study results in the U.S.

For the moment, U.S. experts are siding with estrogen, arguing that "for every woman who might lose her life to breast cancer because of long-term estrogen use, another seven or eight might be spared from premature death by heart attack or stroke."

Using prescription records, researchers identified 23,244 menopausal women taking estrogen and then compared the names with those of breast-cancer patients appearing in the national Cancer Registry. (In Sweden, physicians must report all newly diagnosed cases of cancer to the registry.)

After matching up the names, researchers compared estrogen brands, dosage and duration of use. Long-term estrogen users had a 10 percent increase in breast-cancer risk, and the risk jumped to 70 percent after nine years of use, researchers said. Estradiol, a potent form of estrogen, was the most commonly prescribed and a higher risk factor than estriols, less potent forms.

Many physicians — already aware of estrogen's link with uterine cancer — prescribe a combination of estrogen and progestin (another hormone) for menopausal patients. Although progestin counteracts estrogen's negative effect on uterine cancer, women on combination therapy are more at risk of developing breast cancer, researchers said.

"Estrogen apparently has a [cancer-causing] effect because it stimulates the growth of cells of the breast and uterine lining ... Progestin counteracts that effect on the uterine cells but acts with estrogen to stimulate breast cell growth ... Progestin might therefore [increase] estrogen's effects on breast cancer."

## Depression affects cancer survival rates

Women with breast cancer who got together in weekly group therapy sessions survived almost twice as long as women who received only regular cancer treatment, Dr. David Spiegel recently told the American Psychiatric Association. In addition to regular medical therapy, the women who lived the longest met weekly in "supportive group therapy," Spiegel says.

He studied 86 women with metastatic breast cancer over a 10-year period. (Metastatic means that the cancer has spread from the original site to another location.) All were receiving standard drug, chemical or radiation treatments.

About half the women participated in group therapy during the first year. Women in the weekly therapy group survived an average of 34.8 months. But women who received conventional medical treatment alone, without the group meetings, survived just an average of 18.9 months, according to Spiegel's study.

"Furthermore, there was a trend linking group attendance with longevity among treatment patients," the doctor says.

These findings match those of other doctors who have found that "secondary depression can actually shorten survival," reports *Medical World News* (30,13:20). "When depression accompanies a medical problem, patients are sicker, need more medication, and spend more days in the hospital," the magazine report says.

Spiegel, an associate professor of psychiatry and behavioral sciences at Stanford University School of Medicine, says he hopes his research will encourage metastatic cancer patients to actively participate in group therapy.

Diagnosing and treating depression in cancer patients can affect the outcome of the disease, according to Dr. Charles Nemeroff in a speech to the American Psychiatric Association. Nemeroff, a professor at Duke University in North Carolina, warns that depression can impair the body's immune system. "The last thing you want in cancer patients is an impaired immune response," Nemeroff said. "We need to aggressively diagnose and treat cancer patients with depression."

## Eating fish may lower breast cancer risk

Women who eat fish regularly may lower their risk of getting breast cancer, according to a preliminary statistical study in the journal *Nutrition and Cancer* (12,1:61).

Researchers at two Canadian cancer institutes analyzed how people eat in 32 countries around the world, including the United States. They looked at each country's average daily intake of total fats, animal fat, meat, cereal, milk, sugar, animal oil, total oils of all kinds, fish, coffee, tea, cocoa and riboflavin (one of the B vitamins). Then they compared peoples' diets with breast cancer rates for those countries.

They found what several other studies have shown — breast cancer rates go up where women eat more fats, especially animal fats. But the new study also indicated that in countries where fish consumption is high, breast cancer rates are lower.

The researchers linked this statistical finding with the possibility that diets with a lot of fish offer some protection against breast cancer. "The observation that percent calories from fish is inversely related to (breast cancer) risk implies a protective role for this dietary component," says the report. They speculated that protection might come from the highly polyunsaturated omega-3 fatty acids contained in many kinds of fish from deep, cold waters.

They noted that very little research has been done before now to see if diets high in omega-3 fatty acids offer some protection against breast cancer. They called for more research to follow up their findings.

The same study also indicated that the rate of atherosclerosis (disease of the arteries caused by build-up of plaques containing fatty cholesterol) is linked in the same way. Where fish consumption (as a percent of total calories consumed) is high, artery disease is lower.

In the past several years, many studies have indicated the beneficial effect omega-3 (popularly known as fish oil) fatty acids have on lowering blood cholesterol levels, as well as a few problems with taking supplements.

For example, some people who take fish oil capsules experience burping and fishy aftertaste. In addition, diabetics and people who are on blood-thinning medicines or aspirin therapy should avoid fish oil supplements unless they have specific permission from their doctor.

Studies are underway to determine omega-3's effect on several other kinds of cancer, as well. In one case, omega-3 supplements given in capsule form seemed to help prevent the spread of cancer cells during and after cancer surgery, according to a Harvard Medical School study.

# Colon Cancer

## Dietary fiber may actively fight cancer

Scientists have discovered an active ingredient in dietary fiber that may help to prevent cancer and treat established cancer. According to the journal *Carcinogenesis* (10,3:625), fiber contains inositol hexaphosphate (InsP6), which was effective in significantly reducing the size and number of colon and rectal cancers in rats and mice.

Inositol hexaphosphate, also known as phytic acid, is found in wheat, corn, oats and rice. It is "an abundant plant seed component present in many, but not all, fiber-rich diets," researchers report in the journal *Cancer* (56,4:717). Until now, doctors knew that dietary fiber helps reduce the risk of cancer, but they believed it was because fiber helps move waste through the body and reduces the amount of time that cancer-causing substances can build up in the colon.

In a recent study, Dr. Abulkalam Shamsuddin of the

University of Maryland in Baltimore removed InsP6 from fiber and gave it to test animals in their drinking water. The test animals otherwise had no extra fiber in their diet. Even without the roughage, "the treated animals developed significantly fewer cancers, and 'their cancers were two-thirds smaller' than those of untreated controls," Dr. Shamsuddin said.

In an earlier study reported in *Carcinogenesis* (9,4:577), he found that inositol hexaphosphate reduced the effects of cancer in the large intestine. Other studies by Graf and Eaton reported in *Cancer* (56,4:717) also showed that InsP6 suppresses colon cancer and other inflammatory bowel diseases.

Shamsuddin decided to study the effects of InsP6 when he noticed that groups with high-fiber diets often had different rates of cancer. The amount of InsP6 in the diet seemed to be the only difference, so he decided to test InsP6's effectiveness without the fiber content.

Since InsP6 and Ins are effective agents against large intestinal cancer "in two different species with two different carcinogens (cancer-causing agents), are found naturally, and have relatively little toxicity, they should therefore be seriously considered in our strategies for prevention" of this cancer in humans, Dr. Shamsuddin reported to the Eighth Annual Meeting of the American Association for Cancer Research.

Tablets or capsules of InsP6 could one day be used in the treatment of human cancer because InsP6 can be extracted easily, he said.

Research by Dr. Lillian Thompson at the University of Toronto has also shown that InsP6 has an anti-cancer effect in mice. Other studies showed that InsP6 given after five months of cancer helped to slow the cancer growth.

"Large intestinal cancer is the second most common cancer in the United States with an expected 147,000 new cases" per year, *Carcinogenesis* reports.

## High-fiber diet slashes rectal cancer rates

A high-fiber diet can slash your risk of rectal cancer, a four-year scientific study indicates. It can do this by reducing the number of non-cancerous tumors of the rectum, according to encouraging results reported in the *Journal of the National Cancer Institute* (81,17:1290).

Best results seemed to happen with dietary fiber levels of nearly one ounce every day. That's about twice what most Americans eat regularly.

The high-fiber diet seems to fight formation of benign rectal polyps. These are little tumors on stalks. Sometimes polyps look like tiny mushrooms growing out of the walls of the rectum and lower intestine.

These benign polyps, if not discovered or if left untreated, almost always turn into cancer, the report says. Previous studies have shown that high-fiber diets decrease risks of getting colon cancer.

So researchers studied 58 people to determine whether they would reap the same benefits farther down the digestive tract.

Before the study began, patients were given a baseline examination to calculate the size and number of polyps. There were three groups: sixteen took vitamin C and vitamin E with a low-fiber supplement (vitamin group), twenty were given the vitamins with a high-fiber supplement (high-fiber group), and 22 received only a low-fiber breakfast cereal supplement (control group).

On the average, the vitamin group took in 11.3 grams of wheat fiber per day; the high-fiber group, 22.4 grams; and the control group, 12.2 grams. One ounce equals just over 28 grams.

Researchers chose wheat fiber and vitamins C and E because they have shown the best results in anticancer studies. The wheat fiber — a non-water-soluble kind of dietary fiber — came from a common brand of breakfast cereal.

Every three months, researchers examined all the groups to see if the number of tumors rose or fell. In addition, nurses counseled people having trouble following the diet.

After six months, polyp size and numbers had been cut in half in the high-fiber group, researchers said. Those who took vitamins with a low-fiber cereal generally broke even — no increase and no decrease in tumors.

"A high prescribed fiber intake and, to a lesser extent, a high vitamin intake, were associated with lower polyp number ratios," according to the report. This is good news, especially for people with a family history of rectal tumors.

Compliance in the study was low, meaning that the people being studied failed to stick strictly to their diets. That surprised the researchers, since the patients were aware of their cancer risk. Compliance was highest overall for the high-fiber group, which also showed the best results, followed by the vitamin group and the control group.

In addition to diet therapy, treating polyps in the colon with nonsteroidal anti-inflammatory drugs (NSAIDs) shows promising results, according to *Medical World News* (30,18:23).

NSAIDs are effective because they limit the production of prostaglandins, a type of fatty acid, high concentrations of which are found in tumors.

Taken daily, a NSAID called indomethacin stopped polyp formation in 11 patients who had already undergone surgery to remove colon tumors. More studies are planned.

## Other natural ways to help protect against colon cancer

The results of a study by researchers from the University of Utah School of Medicine say, that of "... the food groups examined, fruit appeared to have the greatest protective effect. High intakes of fruits and vegetables had a beneficial effect on the colon."

Other studies in the *Journal of the National Cancer Institute* (55:15) and the *Journal of Epidemiology* (109:132) have shown a direct link between high fiber and a lower incidence of colon cancer. Despite those findings, doctors were not sure what type of fiber was most effective.

For this study, the Utah team evaluated "various types and sources of fiber in the diet" of more than 500 men and women for five years. Crude fiber was the most important fiber-type in the study, as it consistently decreased the risk of colon cancer in both men and women.

The average person consumes "only 15 to 20 grams of fiber a day, when they need 25 to 40 grams," according to Dr. Denis Burkitt, one of the most respected researchers in the field of dietary fiber.

By increasing daily intake of soluble fiber and insoluble fiber to at least 25 grams, adults and children can help prevent colon cancer as well as "digestive disorders such as constipation, irritable bowel syndrome (IBS), hemorrhoids, and diverticular disease," Dr. Burkitt said.

Soluble fiber, like pectin in apples, is easily dissolved in water. Soluble fiber bonds chemically with certain substances like cholesterol and moves them quickly through the digestive tract.

Insoluble fiber, like cellulose (in whole grains) and hemicellulose (in vegetables) doesn't dissolve in water. Instead such fiber absorbs water like a sponge, softening waste products in the intestines and speeding it out of the body.

Both kinds of fiber are needed for healthy digestion.

In addition to crude fiber, fruits and vegetables, another natural ingredient — ash — seems to provide protection against colon cancer, according to a new study in the *Journal of the National Cancer Institute* (80,18:1474). Ash is defined as "the mineral residue after all the combustible (burnable) components of food samples have been removed."

Calcium, which is a major component of ash, was also found "to have a strong dose-response protective effect against colon cancer." That means the protective effect went up as the dose went up.

## Does colon cancer thrive where the sun doesn't shine?

To protect yourself from colon cancer, get more winter sunshine, a new study suggests.

For several years now, scientists have noticed that colon cancer rates are higher in parts of the world that receive less sunshine.

In fact, a recent government study shows that the highest death rates from colon cancer occur along a line from Maine to Iowa.

Six researchers in Maryland and California wondered if the unexplained differences might be related to the "sunshine" vitamin — vitamin D.

They looked at blood levels of vitamin D among some of the 25,620 volunteers tested in a Maryland county in 1974. After nine years, the researchers checked back to see who had come down with colon cancer out of that group.

They found that people with blood concentrations of 20 nanograms of vitamin D per milliliter or higher were three times less likely to develop colon cancer. (A nanogram is one-billionth of a gram.)

People with lower levels of activated vitamin D were at greater risk for colon cancer, indicates the report in *The Lancet* (2, 8673:1178), a British medical publication.

Vitamin D levels in the blood vary from season to season, especially in colder climates that receive fewer hours of sunlight. Sun rays activate a forerunner of vitamin D in the skin and turn it into a form that's usable by body tissues.

In Britain, vitamin D levels in blood vary from an average of about 13 nanograms per milliliter in March to over 20 nanograms per milliliter in August, according to the *Lancet* report.

In elderly British people, winter vitamin D blood levels were even lower — in some cases one-sixth the summer levels, the report says.

They apparently were not getting enough sunshine, as well as not getting enough of the activated form of vitamin D through supplements.

"Anything that blocks sunshine from penetrating the skin will reduce the amount of vitamin D that the body makes," according to *Vitamin and Mineral Encyclopedia* (FC&A Publishing, 1987: pg. 48).

It's the ultra-violet rays that trigger the vitamin D into action in the body.

Since recent reports have urged people to avoid sunburns or too much ultra-violet exposure for fear of higher skin cancer rates, here's a case for moderation.

The body needs some ultra-violet rays to activate needed vitamin D, but not so much sunshine exposure that it would harm the skin.

Generally speaking, the study suggests that people should try to get more sunshine during autumn and winter months to keep blood levels of vitamin D closer to summer levels.

"The ultra-violet rays only penetrate the atmosphere when

the sun is very high on the horizon," says the Encyclopedia. "Very little ultra-violet light reaches the earth's surface in northern latitudes in the winter months even when the sun is at its highest point at mid-day."

But just a few minutes of mid-day sun exposure during the summer produces all the vitamin D the body can use, the book says.

A caution — don't overdo the sun seeking. Only a little activated vitamin D over the recommended dietary allowance (RDA) can produce side effects ranging from mild (headache, ringing of the ears, nausea) to severe (damage to heart and kidneys, even death).

Many of the unpleasant effects of sunburn are really caused by vitamin D overdose, says the *Encyclopedia.*

The study also indicates that calcium, especially in milk products, seems to help vitamin D lower the risk of cancer of the colon.

"Of all the nutrients analyzed ... (including fat, total calorie intake and dietary fiber), only vitamin D and calcium affected the incidence of colon cancer," the *Lancet* study reports.

According to several other studies, other protections against colon cancer include fresh fruits, fresh vegetables and healthy amounts of dietary fiber.

Colon and rectal cancers kill 55,000 Americans a year, most of them over age 50, according to a report from the Centers for Disease Control.

Four of every 10 deaths occur in the 60 to 74 age bracket, and another four of 10 occur in the 75 and older bracket, the

CDC says.

It's the second leading cause of cancer death among men and the third leading cancer killer among women.

The moral is clear: if you can't get much sunshine, ask your doctor about getting your activated vitamin D by drinking vitamin-D-supplemented milk or by taking vitamin D tablets. However, don't take extra vitamin D without checking with your doctor first.

# Mouth Cancer

## Raw fruit lowers oral cancer risk

Cancer of the mouth is a devastating, disfiguring disease thought by many researchers to be linked to smoking, especially pipes, and use of chewing tobacco and snuff. It usually starts as a red or thickened white patch or a painless ulcer inside the mouth. The abnormal area, known as a lesion, is most common on the lips, tongue and floor of the mouth.

Cancer of the mouth and throat ranks number six on the most-common-cancer list among men and women combined. But men over 45 are twice as likely as women to develop it. Some forms of oral cancer are increasing in the U.S., due to the popularity of chewing and smokeless tobacco among younger men, says a report in *The Lancet* (2,8658:311).

Although lip cancer is detected easily (and treated more successfully than mouth cancer), most people wait too long before seeing a doctor. Long delays before treatment usually mean that the single, local cancer has spread to other areas. The big delay results in a five-year survival rate of only 30 percent.

Oral cancer is preventable, if you observe the following guidelines:

(1) stop smoking,
(2) decrease your alcohol intake
(3) and improve diet and oral hygiene.

See your dentist regularly because oral cancer screening is part of a routine dental examination.

Now there's also news from a recent report from the National Cancer Institute that indicates if you eat more raw fruit you may lower your risk of getting cancers of the mouth and throat.

NCI researchers say that vitamin C, carotene and fiber present in generous amounts in raw fruits may be part of the reason for the protection, but not the only reason. They failed to find a similar preventive effect in vegetables, some of which also contain those same nutritional ingredients.

The study says that people eating more than four raw fruit servings every day have about half the oral cancer risk of people who average eating one or fewer servings daily. The researchers think the extra anti-cancer action may be due to the mechanical cleansing action of the raw fruit during chewing and swallowing. Another reason might be the presence in fruit of ellagic acid, thought to be a cancer inhibitor.

Just eating some cooked vegetables without fruit failed to lower the risk of oral cancers. But chewing crispy vegetables did have a beneficial effect, but not as much good effect as the multiple servings of raw fruit each day.

The same study says that drinking coffee and other hot beverages has no effect, either positive or negative, on mouth and throat cancer risks.

## Vitamin A may prevent oral cancer

A recent study indicates that taking vitamin A or its "previtamin" form, beta carotene, may reduce the risk of getting oral cancer, even among heavy users of tobacco.

Scientists from the British Columbia Cancer Research Center in Vancouver gave weekly doses of 200,000 international units (IU) of vitamin A to 21 persons in a study in India. The persons studied all chewed tobacco mixtures and showed signs of developing oral cancers.

The treatment shrunk precancerous white spots (called leukoplakias) on the tongue and mucous lining of the mouth in 12 of the persons studied. The vitamin therapy also prevented new sores from forming during the year-long study. That degree of prevention over such a long period impressed the researchers, the report said.

The researchers worried about the possible toxic effects of megadoses of vitamin A over a year's time. Vitamin A is fat-soluble and is stored by the body. (On the other hand, vitamin C, which is water-soluble, passes quickly through the body and must be replenished daily.)

Continued overdoses of vitamin A can lead to serious

health problems. To compare the vitamin doses involved, remember that the U.S. minimum dietary requirements of vitamin A for an adult add up to 35,000 IU in a week's time. The Indian patients received more than five times that amount every week.

The Vancouver scientists are looking for ways to avoid the overdose danger and still get the cancer prevention effects. One way, now being studied, may be to take smaller "maintenance" doses of vitamin A, the report said. Another may be to eat red palm oil, which is rich in beta carotene, the study said.

Using beta carotene to prevent oral cancer shows promising results in other research as well. A report on a study of beta carotene benefits was recently presented to the American Society of Clinical Oncology at a meeting in San Francisco, says *Medical World News* (30,16:19).

In the study, each of 23 people with precancerous patches in their mouths received a 30-milligram daily dose of beta carotene. Within six months, the beta carotene treatment apparently caused the sore-like areas to shrink by half in 17 of the 23 people.

Beta carotene is a yellowish substance that the body converts into true vitamin A. You can reap beta carotene's anti-cancer benefits by eating more leafy, dark-green vegetables and deep-yellow fruits such as kale, spinach, carrots, peaches, papayas and cantaloupe, according to *Medical World News*. Normal servings of these sources can provide five to six milligrams of beta carotene daily. That allows your body to produce about one milligram of vitamin A, which is within the range recommended for good health, according to *The Merck Manual* (15th edition, pg. 900).

Previous studies have found that vitamin A-type compounds seem to fight formation of several kinds of cancers, including those of the larynx (voice box), esophagus, stomach and bladder. Ongoing studies are measuring beta carotene's potential for preventing lung and skin cancers.

# Pancreatic Cancer

## Amazing fish oil fights deadly cancer of the pancreas

New research suggests that a diet high in fish oil may do double duty in fighting cancer of the pancreas. First, the omega-3 fatty acid in the fish oil seems to prevent the formation of precancerous tumors, based on animal studies reported in *Science News* (35,25:390).

Second, the oil — from a common deep-sea fish called menhaden — also may hinder the spread of a tumor that's already turned into cancer.

Cancer of the pancreas is the fifth leading cancer killer in the United States. Scientists suspect that high-fat diets are a major risk factor for getting this disease. The pancreas is a banana-sized gland behind the stomach that produces digestive juices and hormones.

Researchers are finding out that what kinds of fats you eat

could make a lot of difference in your cancer risk. For example, in one animal study, rats were injected with a powerful chemical that is known to trigger pancreatic cancer. The rats then were fed a high-fat diet containing either 20 percent corn oil or 20 percent fish oil, according to a report of the study published in the *Journal of the National Cancer Institute* (81,11:858).

The rats fed fish oil developed only about one-third as many precancerous tumors as the corn oil-fed rats, the report says. After tumors turned into cancer, the researchers were able to slow their growth and spread by lowering the total amount of fat in the diets.

"We are showing that using different (dietary fats), you can affect the progression of a cancer," says biochemist Reuven Reich in the *SN* report.

Other studies suggest that omega-3 (the short name for eicosapentanoic acid, found in abundance in cold water fish) itself slows down the spread of cancer cells from their original site to other parts of the body.

"There's no doubt about it. Something about fish oil puts it in a separate category from the average oil," agrees Leonard Cohen of the American Health Foundation in Valhalla, N.Y. But, he notes, you have to eat a "hefty" amount before seeing the anti-cancer effects.

How much omega-3 should be eaten daily is still up in the air. One recent nutrition study suggests that the government should develop a recommended minimum daily dietary amount for average Americans. No such MDA (minimum daily allowance) for omega-3 currently exists.

Many doctors recommend that you get the benefits of

omega-3 oil by eating cold water fish rather than by taking capsule supplements containing fish oil.

People with diabetes and those who take aspirin or blood thinners or have recently had surgery should be especially careful about taking fish oil supplements. The omega-3 acts like a blood thinner itself. Such combinations of blood thinners and fish oil could cause excessive bleeding.

# Skin Cancer

## Risk factors for skin cancer

Although anyone can develop a skin cancer, some people are more susceptible than others. You should be especially careful about protecting yourself or loved ones from the harmful effect of the sun if you have one or more of the following risks, warns The Skin Cancer Foundation:

- Fair skin and/or freckles
- Blond, red or light-brown hair
- Blue, green or gray eyes
- A tendency to burn easily and to tan little or not at all
- A tendency to burn before tanning
- A family history of skin cancer
- Residence in a warm, sunny climate
- Long periods of daily exposure or short periods of intense exposure

• A large number of moles

## A way to calculate your skin cancer risk

More people than ever are developing new cases of melanoma, and more people than ever are dying of the rapidly spreading cancer. Skin moles have long been considered to be a major signal of a high risk of skin cancer. The more moles on a person's body, the greater the cancer risk, doctors have believed. Doctors have relied upon counts of moles on the arms or the whole body to gauge a person's risk.

Now we are told that the people at greatest risk for melanoma are those with many skin moles on one particular area of the body — their lower legs, according to a new study published in the *Journal of the National Cancer Institute* (81,12:948). In fact, if you have 10 or more moles of any type below your knees, you face four times the risk of melanoma compared with a person who has 10 or more moles on the arms, the study says.

People with 12 or more moles on their lower legs were twice as likely to develop melanoma as people with 27 or more arm moles, the study says. Even small numbers of leg moles had a higher prediction rate for cancer than the same number of arm moles. "The relative risk associated with one to nine lower (leg) moles was twice that associated with one to nine arm moles," the researchers report. They counted both raised and flat types of moles to get the clinical figures.

Researcher and dermatologist Martin A. Weinstock wasn't sure why moles on the lower legs were such a powerful marker for increased rates of skin cancer. But he noted that having a concentration of moles in a particular spot on the body didn't necessarily mean that skin cancer would crop up in or near that spot. Instead, a skin cancer was just as likely to develop somewhere else on the body, away from a cluster of moles.

The study also shifted blame for skin cancer away from the moles themselves. "This study suggests it's not the moles themselves that cause melanoma," according to a report in *Science News* (136,2:30). "Rather, (Weinstock) says, they serve as a sentinel of who stands in especially high risk."

One problem for mole counters, even medical experts, is accurately identifying the several different kinds of moles. Three skin specialists report in the *British Medical Journal* (298,6690:16) that even experienced doctors may miss or misdiagnose half of all cancerous and non-cancerous moles. Their report indicates that in only half the cases did all three doctors agree in their diagnoses of colored (pigmented) moles, including cancerous types.

One kind of mole — dysplastic naevus — is an especially high risk signal for skin cancer. The three British doctors say that, as a group, they identified these moles correctly only 51 percent of the time. "Of greater importance is the ability, or inability, to recognize dysplastic naevi," the doctors write. "Only 20 (51 percent) out of 39 dysplastic naevi were identified correctly by all (three) observers, whereas 24 (harmless) lesions were thought to be dysplastic on clinical grounds."

Such remarkable honesty on the part of experienced skin specialists indicates that it may be wise to seek more than one doctor's opinion if you have a question about your moles.

## A serious warning from your fingernails

If you see a widening band of color running up and down your fingernail, you might need to see a doctor right away, according to a professor of medicine at the University of Mississippi Medical Center.

That colored band could be an early signal of a rapid-spreading skin cancer, the doctor says in *Modern Medicine* (57,5:57).

Two practicing physicians suggest in the medical journal that you may want to become better acquainted with your fingernails and toenails.

Those lowly parts may serve as important early warning signs for several serious ailments, including liver and kidney failure, heart and blood vessel disorders, poisonings, various painful inflammations of the joints and muscles, and a deadly form of skin cancer called melanoma.

"Melanoma does appear in the nail unit," according to Dr. Ralph Daniel III, clinical associate professor of dermatology at the Jackson school. "If you see a widening brownish or blackish band running up and down the nail, especially in a person of middle age or older, a biopsy may be indicated."

Daniel suggests that you get your nails carefully examined by a doctor every time you have a physical examination.

"Lines or changes in nail coloration may indicate disease

or exposure to toxic substances in the home or workplace," the *Modern Medicine* report says.

Pits and beads on nails also may provide clues to the presence of rheumatoid arthritis and two kinds of muscular inflammations called fibromyalgia and myofascial syndromes.

Out of 150 patients suffering from myofascial syndrome, 122 had nail pits and 76 had nail beads. Of 93 patients with fibromyalgia, 80 had nail pits and 45 had beads on their nail surfaces, according to Dr. Kip L. Kemple of Portland, Ore.

In addition, 25 out of 30 patients with rheumatoid arthritis also had beads on their nails, "a surprising association," according to the report in *Modern Medicine*.

Other nail signs include the following:

**Double white horizontal lines** — may be sign of liver disease or poor nutrition.

**Spoon nails** — the nail surface forms a cup or depression. May be sign of iron deficiency or anemia.

**Yellow nails** — hard, yellow nails may be sign of chronic lung disease like emphysema or chronic bronchitis, or it could be sinus trouble.

**Half-brown, half-normal nails** — could be sign of serious kidney trouble if the nail half nearest the knuckle is normal but the half toward the end of the nails is brownish.

**Club nails** — the opposite of spoon nails, the nail is raised

147

abnormally high with steep side curves. May be signal of heart failure, lung disease or thyroid problems.

**Dark specks on the nail bed** — known as splinter hemorrhages, these could be harmless. But beware if the specks cluster at the nail end nearest the knuckle and show up in several nails at once. These could be early signs of a bacterial infection of a heart valve, a serious condition that needs to be treated with antibiotics.

**Soft nails** — normally harmless. Occasionally, it could indicate an overactive thyroid gland.

**Brittle nails** — usually caused by detergents or nail polish remover. Once in a while, it's a sign of an underactive thyroid gland.

Although he's done only preliminary statistical work on the association between nails and bodily diseases, Dr. Kemple says the nail signs may be a marker for whole groups of "systemic biologic disturbances."

At each physical, Dr. Daniel says, the nails should be examined in a good light.

The toes should be relaxed and any nail polishes or coatings should be removed before the exam, the doctor says. "To localize any discoloration, shine a penlight up through the finger or toe," Daniel recommends.

# Vitamin product prevents skin cancer

We know that the best way to prevent skin cancer is to avoid exposure to ultraviolet (UV) rays from the sun and in places like tanning booths. But some people at high risk may need to take further preventive action, doctors at Boston University School of Medicine report.

Five people with a rare skin disorder (xeroderma pigmentosum) that causes cancer took high doses of Accutane® for two years. Researchers found that it completely prevented the development of skin cancer, according to the *New England Journal of Medicine* (318:25).

Accutane® (generic name isotretinoin) is a strong, toxic derivative of vitamin A that is used to treat severe cases of disfiguring acne. It causes birth defects in pregnant women and is considered a drug of "last resort" in acne patients because of its serious side effects. The study said the researchers believe that if Accutane® can prevent skin cancer, even in such a small study, some less poisonous form of vitamin A may be found that also can prevent the disease. The search is underway.

The good news for light-skinned persons or those with a family history of skin cancer is that the vitamin A-derivative approach is not just a treatment; it represents actual prevention of skin cancer among high-risk people.

Regular vitamin A is an absolutely essential part of a normal diet, necessary for eye health and good vision, especially at night. It helps the body resist respiratory diseases and shortens durations of several diseases. In normal amounts, it aids in keeping outer layers of tissues and organs healthy and promotes normal growth and strong bones.

Although the body stores vitamin A, men need about 5,000 international units (IUs) to prevent deficiencies; women require about 4,000 IUs daily. Some of the best natural sources include fish liver oil, liver, carrots (one cup of cooked, diced carrots contains about 15,000 IUs of vitamin A), green and yellow vegetables, yellow fruits, eggs, milk, and dairy products.

Don't take too much vitamin A. Daily megadoses of vitamin A of 100,000 IUs taken for several months can produce poisonous side effects.

## Sun exposure guidelines

- Use a sunscreen with a SPF (sun protection factor) of at least 15.
- Follow the label directions.
- Test the sunscreen on a small patch of skin to see if any irritation occurs.
- Apply sunscreen 30 minutes before exposure to the sun. Remember that even on cloudy days, up to 80 percent of the sun's radiation reaches the ground.
- Apply sunscreen to clean, dry skin.
- Apply it evenly and thickly over your entire body — remembering your lips, ears, hands, forearms and the back of the neck, all of which are high exposure areas.
- Reapply sunscreen after swimming or sweating.

- Avoid direct sunlight between 10 a.m. and 3 p.m.
- Remember that ultraviolet rays can penetrate through loosely woven or wet clothes. Wear sunscreen under your clothes when necessary.
- Be especially careful at higher altitudes, or when you are closer to the equator because the sun's rays are stronger.
- Watch for any changes in your skin — new raised growths, itchy patches, non-healing sores, changes in moles or new colored areas — and report them to your doctor immediately.

Sources: *The Skin Cancer Foundation, U.S. Pharmacist* (14,4:27) and *Natural Remedies for Super Perfect Health* (FC&A Publishing).

## Why sunscreens don't always work

Allergies, photosensitivity, or improper application may make sunscreens ineffective and increase the risk of skin cancer, aging spots, wrinkles, redness, rash or skin irritation.

Benzophenone, a chemical used in high-protection sunscreens, may cause allergic dermatitis in sensitive people, dermatologist Elizabeth Knobler reports in *Modern Medicine* (57,3:49). Redness and itching can occur either when the skin is exposed to the sun or just from contact with benzophenone. "Because sunscreen formulations may vary from year to year (even though product names remain the same)," Dr. Knobler recommends reading the product label and avoiding sunscreens containing benzophenone.

Photosensitivity is an exaggerated reaction to sunlight. It

can be caused by using certain drugs, cosmetics, or perfumes, according to *Patient Care* (6:15). Redness, swelling, hives and itching are symptoms of photosensitivity. If your skin is photosensitive, it reacts to the sun more quickly and more severely than normal skin.

Some of the drugs that can lead to photosensitivity are Retin-A, thiazide diuretics ("water pills" used in treating high blood pressure), tetracycline, antidiabetics, psoralens, oral contraceptives, antipsychotics, antidepressants, antihistamines, antibacterials, anticancer drugs, and corticosteroids.

Coal tar products, coal tar dyes, musk fragrances, and some other perfumes also can cause photosensitivity, according to *Patient Care*. People taking these drugs or using coal tar products should avoid or limit their exposure to sun. When exposure is unavoidable, the strongest possible sunscreen should be used.

Even eating some foods can bring a reaction. Limes, celery, lemons, parsley, and certain oranges can cause photosensitivity, Dr. Jonathan Held reports in the *American Family Physician* (39,4:143).

If the skin is exposed to one of these fruits or vegetables and then the ultraviolet rays of the sun, a severe skin irritation may occur. The irritation may take the form of redness, itching and rash. Redness and blistering usually appear about 48 hours after exposure, Held warns.

Grocery workers are especially vulnerable to this type of skin irritation. They should be careful to avoid direct contact with limes, celery, lemons, parsley and bergamot oranges.

Sunscreens can be harmful to some people who have a photosensitive reaction to the sun caused by a particular form of ultraviolet light known as ultraviolet A. The reaction is known as polymorphic light eruption. According to *The Lancet* (1,8635:429), "between 14 percent and 28 percent of the adult female population" suffers some form of this skin reaction.

Since most sunscreens only protect against the ultraviolet B rays, the researchers warn that using a sunscreen is dangerous for these sensitive people. The sunscreen will block the ultraviolet B rays but actually will allow more exposure to ultraviolet A rays. That extra exposure will increase the redness and itching that occurs. "Patients with polymorphic light eruption ... should be advised to sunbathe without sunscreens but only for a short time," according to *The Lancet*.

Sunscreens containing PABA (para-aminobenzoic acid) or alcohol can also cause irritation in sensitive people. To avoid an unwanted allergic reaction, apply your sunscreen to a small area of skin and watch for any unusual irritation. Try this test at least 24 hours before using the sunscreen on your whole body.

Even if you do not have an allergic or photosensitive reaction, you need to be "sun smart" to reduce your risk of skin cancer, wrinkles and age spots. Use a sunscreen of at least 15 SPF (sun protection factor) daily, especially on your nose, hands and face. However, avoid the problem ones outlined above. The SPF reading tells you how much extra protection you have from the ultraviolet rays. For example, an SPF of 15 means you have 15 times more protection than without the sunscreen.

Use a thick application of sunscreen. The *U.S. Pharmacist* explains that a sunscreen must be applied thickly — at the same thickness that the sunscreen was tested at — for it to be as effective as its rating number. "To achieve a good protection from the sun, a layer thickness of 2 milligrams per square centimeter is often recommended," the journal says. However, a recent study found that most people only applied half that amount — reducing their sunscreen protection level by half.

Avoid artificial tanning methods. Learn to accept the fact that untanned skin is healthier than the "tanned" look.

Be aware that other irritants also may affect your skin. Some of those irritants may be in your jewelry box. For that reason, avoid olive wood products, especially jewelry made with olive wood. Many people with sensitive skin will experience an allergic reaction to olive wood, *Cutis* (43,3:202) reports.

Besides jewelry, olive wood is often made into napkin rings, walking sticks, knife handles, musical instruments, and crucifixes. All of those can cause redness, itching and swelling upon contact with the skin. The skin reaction usually ends when contact with the olive wood is stopped, the journal report says.

# Cholesterol

## The cholesterol controversy

Millions of Americans have been confused by the recent controversy regarding cholesterol. Can cutting cholesterol really help you live longer? Or is it an overblown myth that has no scientific basis?

*Nutrition Action,* a newsletter that is published by the Center for Science in the Public Interest, has asked experts on heart disease to respond to that allegation. These experts say that many factors do indeed contribute to heart and artery disease: heredity, smoking, high blood pressure, diabetes, lack of exercise, and being overweight. But the fact also remains that heart disease is a problem only in those countries where the typical diet is high in cholesterol.

There is no getting around the fact that for every one

percent reduction in serum cholesterol in the blood there is a two percent to four percent reduction in the risk of heart attack. And it's difficult to ignore the famous Framingham Heart Study, based on 5,200 residents of Framingham, Massachusetts.

It shows that high levels of LDL (low-density lipoprotein) and low levels of HDL (high-density lipoprotein) place the elderly at greater risk of heart attack. It has also shown that after menopause, blood cholesterol levels are clear indicators of coronary risk for women.

Dr. August Watanabe, chairman of the International Scientific meeting of the American Heart Association, stated in an article in the *Saturday Evening Post* (March, 1989), "The recent data regarding cholesterol pretty convincingly show that it is an important risk factor, and that if you lower the cholesterol you'll reduce the risk for cardiovascular disease … I think it's important for the public to be aware that we are making substantial progress in decreasing mortality from cardiovascular disease. This is very different from any other major category of disease. One reason is better awareness by the public of risk factors such as smoking, dietary factors, cholesterol, etc. I think there is generally a better awareness and people are changing their lifestyles."

True, there is a minority of respected researchers and physicians who question the value of cholesterol reduction in preserving health and preserving life. But, since progress is being made against heart disease, the nation's number one killer, and since reducing cholesterol is a big factor in that progress, it seems unwise to abandon these facts.

The writers of this book hope that you will remember that prevailing scientific evidence is in favor of cholesterol reduction, that many people are healthier today because they are careful about their diets, and that heart disease is something you *can* do something about.

## The facts about cholesterol

Estimates from the National Institutes of Health show that about 40 million Americans have levels of cholesterol high enough to substantially increase their risk of heart and artery disease.

The first step in reducing the risk of heart and artery disease is to have your cholesterol level checked.

A recent survey by the Centers for Disease Control in Atlanta reports that "only 47 percent of persons surveyed have ever had a blood cholesterol level measured, only 19 percent have ever been told their cholesterol level, and only 6 percent actually know their blood cholesterol level."

The National Cholesterol Education Program recommends that every adult should have a total blood cholesterol level measurement at least once every five years.

Until recently it was thought that if your total cholesterol level was below 200 milligrams per deciliter (mg/dl), you would not need another test. The following guidelines have been the accepted standard:

| Total cholesterol levels | Guidelines |
|---|---|
| less than 200 mg/dl<br>200 to 239 mg/dl<br>240 mg/dl and over | desirable<br>borderline high<br>high |
| **LDL-cholesterol levels** | **Guidelines** |
| less than 130 mg/dl<br>130 to 159<br>160 mg/dl and over | desirable<br>borderline high<br>high |
| **HDL-cholesterol levels** | **Guidelines** |
| less than 35 mg/dl | too low |

Source: *Western Journal of Medicine* (150,3:562)

However, a large number of patients whose total cholesterol levels were considered "safe" have been found to have diseased heart arteries, researchers at the Johns Hopkins Medical Institutions in Baltimore report. This discovery has prompted the scientists to question whether current guidelines, issued in October 1987, may need revision.

The scientists evaluated the blood lipid (fat) content of 1,000 patients who had undergone diagnostic coronary angiography, an X-ray of their heart arteries, to search for obstacles that might interfere with blood flow to the heart. Of the 1,000 patients, there were 185 men and four women who had coronary artery disease, even though their total cholesterol levels were less than 200, well within the so-called "desirable" range. Patients with a recent heart attack were excluded from the study because the heart attack would have altered their lipid levels. This left 138 men and three women in the investigation.

Sixty-eight percent of the men and 32 percent of the women had HDL-cholesterol levels of less than 35 milligrams per deciliter. Earlier studies have shown that the risk of heart disease increases as the HDL levels fall. An HDL level of 35 translates into a 50 percent higher risk than an HDL level of 45, according to the Framingham Heart Study. We "were curious to find out if, in fact, there were lipid abnormalities that were prevalent in a patient group that otherwise would not be detected by the present guidelines," said Dr. Michael Miller, one of the researchers.

Medical statistics show, and the Johns Hopkins study confirms, that a low HDL level is a strong predictor of coronary heart disease — even better, some scientists believe, than the presence of high levels of LDL. Scientists believe that HDL helps lower the risk of heart disease by transporting cholesterol to the liver to be processed for excretion.

LDL is one category of cholesterol that many doctors usually term the "bad" cholesterol. It circulates in the blood, depositing fat and cholesterol in the tissues, contributing to the build-up of plaque in the artery wall. This can lead to "hardening" or narrowing of the arteries and increases the risk for high blood pressure and heart problems.

Regardless of their total cholesterol level, doctors should measure and analyze the fasting blood levels of total cholesterol, HDL cholesterol and triglycerides of everyone with heart disease, the researchers recommend. Cholesterol levels of 245 mg/dl were associated with "a twofold greater risk of dying of coronary artery disease in six years," in the Multiple Risk Factor Intervention Trial. Total cholesterol levels of 300 mg/dl quadrupled the risk.

According to Miller, one way to increase HDL levels is to lose weight, particularly for obese patients. If you lose weight, not only will your HDL levels go up, but your triglyceride levels may go down. (Some researchers think that high triglyceride levels in the blood may also be a risk factor for heart disease.) Weight loss also reduces the risk of diabetes, which is itself a contributing factor to heart disease. Regular exercise and quitting smoking will also help to raise HDL levels.

Dietary changes commonly reduce blood cholesterol levels. Polyunsaturated fats, such as those in corn or safflower oil, decrease total cholesterol levels, but they also lower HDL levels. However, Miller says recent studies have shown that monounsaturated fats, such as olive oil, will reduce the total cholesterol without adversely affecting the HDL level.

A recent study by the Centers for Disease Control in Atlanta found that between the ages of 20 and 60 years, men's cholesterol levels increase an average of 50 points. In that same period, women's increase about 70 points. The researchers hope this discovery will help alert younger adults to their future risk of heart disease, so they can choose a healthy diet and lifestyle at an early age.

# "Natural" menopause and high cholesterol

Postmenopausal women have higher cholesterol levels — and greater heart-disease risk — than premenopausal women, says a recent report in *New England Journal of Medicine* (321,10:641). These findings confirm the importance of middle-aged women watching their fat intake.

Natural menopause (without hormone-replacement therapy) leads to an increase in low-density lipoprotein (LDL, or "bad") cholesterol levels and a decrease in high-density lipoprotein (HDL, or "good") cholesterol levels that "exceed those caused by aging," Pittsburgh researchers said. These changes may increase the heart-disease risk for postmenopausal women.

Researchers began their five-year study of premenopausal women in 1983. By 1988, 100 of 541 women had been menopausal for at least one year; 32 received hormone-replacement therapy for about eight months before reevaluation. The "natural menopause" group (69 women) and the hormone-replacement group were matched with an equal number controls, for a total of 202 women in four groups. Of the 32 women on hormone-replacement therapy, three were taking estrogen, five were taking progestogen, and the remainder were taking a combination of those two hormones.

Before the study began, researchers took baseline blood tests to measure insulin levels, triglycerides (a form of fat in the bloodstream) and HDL and LDL cholesterol levels. They also assessed other factors, such as diet, weight, exercise, smoking, alcohol consumption and blood pressure. When a woman had stopped menstruating for one year or had stopped menstruating and received hormone-replacement therapy for a combined total of one year, she was evaluated again and assigned a premenopausal control of the same age and risk factors.

The average age of all participants was 47, and the average duration between examination was two and a half years.

Researchers pinpointed several differences among the natural menopause group even before menopause began. They had significantly higher triglyceride and cholesterol levels than the hormone-replacement group and controls. They were also heavier and smoked more than their own control group.

The natural menopause women had higher [cholesterol and triglyceride] levels "than their premenopausal controls, even at the base-line examination, when all the women were premenopausal. The HDL cholesterol level declined, while the LDL cholesterol level increased." The HDL level did not change in the control group, which also had a smaller increase in LDL cholesterol.

The hormone-replacement group showed no change in insulin and cholesterol levels, but triglycerides increased significantly. "Hormone-replacement therapy may protect against LDL increase but results in a remarkable increase in the triglyceride level," researchers said.

The other factors (diet, exercise, blood pressure) did not affect the study results.

# How effective is high-cholesterol treatment?

People with high cholesterol do not respond equally well to cholesterol-lowering treatment (whether diet or drugs), say New Hampshire researchers, who advocate individual treatment for every patient.

According to a report in *Archives of Internal Medicine* (149,9:1981), the New Hampshire researchers evaluated data from several high-cholesterol studies and noted these trends:

- Elderly men benefited less from high-cholesterol treatment than younger men. Age might influence the response to drug therapy and dietary change, researchers said.
- Smokers do not respond as well as nonsmokers, for the same reasons as cited above.
- The data for men and women are conflicting. Some studies show men at greater risk, while others show women at greater risk.
- Lowering cholesterol benefits people who have high blood pressure more than people with normal blood pressure.
- "The presence of each additional risk factor [for example, obesity and high blood pressure] increases the risk of heart disease by 50 percent to 100 percent," researchers said. Risk factors vary from population to population.
- Overweight, middle-aged men who have a family history

of heart disease should be screened for high cholesterol.

Researchers also point out that cholesterol treatment has a price. "For most Americans, dietary intervention requires substantial and possibly life-long changes in eating habits. Drug therapy requires long-term compliance, is costly, and may produce unpleasant side effects."

## Pros and cons of new cholesterol drug

A new drug to lower cholesterol, Mevacor, has been very successful, but also controversial. For one thing it is very expensive (over a dollar a pill). It also can have side effects on the liver, so the functions of the liver should be monitored regularly.

Dr. Kenneth Cooper, who wrote the best-selling book *Controlling Cholesterol,* was asked recently to comment on using the drug Mevacor to lower cholesterol.

He responded that he uses the drug quite regularly but only on people who have had bypass surgery, who have had heart attacks, and who are not responding to anything else.

Dr. Cooper adds that his best success is when a person takes a 20 milligram tablet at night right before he goes to bed. That tends to slow down the production of the LDL cholesterol that occurs about 3:00 A.M. Dr. Cooper says that researchers at the University of Texas Southwestern Medical School have found that the body produces most of its LDL cholesterol about 3:00 A.M.

If a person can't take the drug at bedtime because of gastric distress, it's just about as good to take one at the evening meal, he adds.

## A vitamin that fights cholesterol

A daily doctor-prescribed supplement of niacin can help lower dangerously high cholesterol levels, according to *Mayo Clinic Nutrition Letter* (2,10:1).

"Daily doses of 0.5 to 6 grams of niacin decrease levels of total cholesterol and LDL [low-density lipoprotein, or "bad"] cholesterol," according to the report.

That's 31 to 375 times the officially recommended daily allowance (RDA) for regular good nutritional purposes.

Niacin, a member of the vitamin B complex, is prescribed in some cases because it stops the production of LDL cholesterol and helps the body absorb carbohydrates.

Experts have known of the vitamin's cholesterol-lowering abilities for more than 30 years and often prescribe it in conjunction with other medications.

In smaller amounts, niacin is found naturally in liver, yeast, lean meat and whole grains.

You might be tempted to self-medicate yourself, but *don't*. The report offers a few reasons:

- When taken in such large doses, niacin acts like a powerful drug and can cause side effects, such as flushing and upset stomach. The higher the dosage, the more severe the side effects. Even 500 milligrams can be very harmful. (Under doctors' orders, timed-release niacin helps control side effects.)

- Niacin is not a cure-all. You must change your diet and increase your exercise to lower cholesterol successfully.
- Your doctor may think that another treatment would work better for you.

In a recent article of the *Saturday Evening Post*, Dr. Kenneth Cooper also warns about the care that must be taken when using niacin to control cholesterol.

He says, "It works in some cases, but you've got to follow patients at least at six-week intervals, because a certain number will develop severe liver problems in conjunction with it. I've hospitalized at least six patients as a result of niacin problems."

## A well-known natural laxative that cuts cholesterol

Millions of people have used a common over-the-counter natural laxative to get relief from occasional constipation. By taking a dietary fiber called psyllium, they likely were helping their hearts at the same time. Psyllium is the main ingredient in laxative products like Metamucil and Fiberall.

Researchers have found that daily doses of just three teaspoons of psyllium can lower cholesterol levels in the blood by 5 percent and can slash levels of "bad" cholesterol by 10 percent or more. The results are in a report in The *Journal of the American Medical Association* (261,23:3419).

For every percentage point you lower your total cholesterol level, your risk of heart attack drops by two percentage points, the report says. In addition, the fiber supplements can raise the proportion of "good" HDL cholesterol while it lowers the "bad" LDL cholesterol. That also fights your risk of heart disease.

The researchers got these results in experiments with people who had mild to moderate cases of hypercholesterolemia, the medical name for too much cholesterol in the blood.

The 75 people had already been put on low-fat diets to treat their condition. Most received some benefit from just that step alone.

In addition to the low-fat diet, half of them took the extra psyllium daily for up to 16 weeks during the experiments. The ones who took the fiber laxative were the ones who had the dramatic additional cuts in cholesterol levels. They took each teaspoonful of psyllium with eight ounces of water.

Besides the beneficial effects of lowering cholesterol, the psyllium supplements had no serious side effects. About one out of six people reported minor discomforts from temporary feelings of fullness with some abdominal cramping. One in 12 had bloating and increased amounts of intestinal gas being passed.

Only one experienced a significant laxative effect. "All of these events were transient and minor in nature, and none required discontinuation of treatment," the *JAMA* article says.

The psyllium fiber worked even better than oat bran,

according to the report. Overall, eight out of 10 people who took the psyllium (in the form of Metamucil) had lower "bad" cholesterol and total cholesterol levels after eight weeks. That compared to almost no changes in the control group, which had been given a fake supplement called a placebo.

Psyllium is the fiber part of seed husks from the common plant, English plantain. The fiber dissolves in water and forms a kind of gel in the digestive system. Doctors still aren't sure *how* the fiber fights cholesterol, only that it does.

Nearly 25 percent of the American adult population — one out of every four of us — has unhealthy cholesterol levels, the study says. Many doctors prefer to use natural means — particularly changes in diet — as the first stage of treatment in lowering blood cholesterol levels.

## A lifestyle change that can reverse heart damage

Diet and lifestyle changes can reverse damage to your heart and arteries, a new study by Dr. Dean Ornish at the University of California, San Francisco confirms.

"Changing your lifestyle can actually begin to reverse coronary blockages," Dr. Ornish told the American Heart Association.

In a year-long study, people with artery problems who practiced meditation, exercised, quit smoking, participated in group counseling and ate a vegetarian diet with less than 10 percent fat, had dramatic improvements in their arteries and cholesterol levels.

However, Ornish warned that a comparison group, which consumed a regular, low-fat diet, just 30 percent fat, who also exercised and quit smoking, did not experience improvement in their arteries — their blockages actually got worse.

Ornish believes that only strict and major lifestyle changes, including stress management techniques, are necessary for drastic improvements in the arteries.

Ornish admits that "there is no way to know for sure" how faithfully the patients followed the strenuous regimen. They are requested to fill out questionnaires, but "the most objective evidence we have that people are following the changes are the striking reductions in total cholesterol and LDL-cholesterol levels, despite the fact that we are not using cholesterol-lowering medications," the scientist explained.

The lifestyle-change group not only experienced a significant decrease in cholesterol levels but also a measurable widening of the coronary arteries that had been narrowed before, Ornish reported.

Total cholesterols declined from a median 227 mg/dl to 136 mg/dl, and the average extent of coronary artery narrowing decreased from 38.8 percent to 34.9 percent.

However, in the control group, there was no significant change in cholesterol levels and the narrowing of the patients' heart arteries continued to get worse, from an average of 44.8 percent to 50.6 percent.

In earlier studies, Ornish had shown that a complete vegetarian diet is needed to help lower LDL (low-density lipoproteins — the harmful cholesterol), *Journal of the American Medical Association* (254:10, 1337-41). A modified vegetarian diet that allowed consumption of dairy products caused unwanted increases in LDL levels.

## Candy bar to lower cholesterol

A cholesterol-lowering drug is now available in a candy bar, known as Cholybar®. Each Cholybar contains four grams of the cholesterol-lowering drug cholestyramine, and up to six bars could be prescribed per day. The chewable "drug" comes in two flavors, raspberry and caramel.

Until Cholybar, cholestyramine was only available as Questran® by Bristol-Myers. Questran is a powder that must be added to water or other fluids before it is taken. Like Cholybar, Questran comes in four-gram increments.

Warner-Lambert, who developed and sells Cholybar, hopes that the candy bar format will make it easier for their patients to take. They think the candy bar will provide the best possible base for the drug to be absorbed by the body.

Cholestyramine can cause bad side effects like constipation, hemorrhoids, abdominal pain, bleeding in the stomach, belching, flatulence, nausea, vomiting, diarrhea, heartburn and loss of appetite. Perhaps the candy bar formulation will help reduce some of these side effects.

Each caramel bar is 18 grams and 50 calories, while the raspberry bars are 22 grams and 60 calories. More flavors are being planned for the future.

However, critics suggest that people who will need to eat several bars per day will be getting too many unneeded calories.

Currently, a prescription is required for Cholybar, and it is only being distributed west of the Rockies. After initial sales in the West are evaluated, and production is increased, Warner-Lambert is hoping to introduce Cholybar throughout the U.S.A.

## Change your eating habits to lower cholesterol

You can make a big change for the better in your blood cholesterol levels just by changing your eating habits. Eating a well-balanced diet is the easiest and least expensive method to reduce cholesterol.

Your goals should be to lower saturated fat intake, which accounts for 40 percent of our daily calorie count. But be careful to keep on getting proper nutrients.

Lower your dietary cholesterol, found in meats, dairy products and animal fats; and count calories. (Fat people are more likely to have higher cholesterol levels than normal-weight people.)

Below are some guidelines to help you choose the healthiest foods to eat.

**Dairy products:** Choose skim milk instead of whole milk; low-fat plain yogurt instead of fruit yogurts made with whole milk; low-fat cheeses (farmer's, mozzarella), and ice milk or sherbet instead of ice cream. Limit egg yolks to less than three per week; use egg whites in place of whole eggs in recipes.

**Meats and seafood:** Think lean. Choose chicken, turkey, and well-trimmed cuts of lean beef. Eat at least two servings of fish per week. Fish from deep, cold waters are best because they're high in essential omega-3 oils. Fresh or frozen fish are better than canned. But if you eat canned fish, choose fish packed in water, not oil.

**Fruits and vegetables:** Eat three servings of fresh fruits daily (except coconuts). Avoid fruit canned in heavy syrup. Read the labels on jams and jellies and choose a low-sugar product. Most vegetables and preparation methods are fine, but avoid avocados, olives, cheese, cream and butter sauces. Restrict starchy vegetables, such as potatoes.

**Cereals, nuts, breads:** Most hot and cold packaged cereals are fine, but watch the sugar and salt content. Also check the labels and buy those that are highest in dietary fiber, vitamins and minerals (remember that *dietary fiber* is not the same thing as *crude fiber*). Use pecans, walnuts and peanuts sparingly. Avoid hydrogenated peanut butter. Choose whole-grain breads, and avoid commercially baked goods, such as cakes and pastries, which are loaded with fat. Instead of egg noodles, choose pastas and rice.

The above guidelines are from *Postgraduate Medicine* and are based on recommendations from the American Heart Association and the National Cholesterol Education Program

Expert Panel.

How you prepare food also will affect your cholesterol levels. You may freely use vinegar, soy sauce (but watch the sodium) and most spices and herbs.

Cooking oils are another matter. Choose polyunsaturated vegetable oils, such as safflower, corn and sesame oils. Avoid lard altogether. Instead of butter, try polyunsaturated margarine instead.

## How to eat less fat

Saturated fats, found in red meats and dairy products, should be reduced to less than 10 percent of total calories. Unsaturated fats, such as fish and vegetable oils, may constitute as much as 10 percent of total calories. Your entire fat intake should be less than one-third of your total daily calories.

- Eliminate or drastically reduce consumption of egg yolks, organ meats and most cheeses.
- Reduce your consumption of butter, bacon, beef, whole milk, cream, chocolate, almost any food of animal origin, hydrogenated vegetable shortenings, coconut oil and palm oil.
- Use monounsaturated oils like olive oil or peanut oil, or polyunsaturated oil like corn, safflower, sesame seed, cottonseed, soybean or sunflower oils. Use soft margarine instead of butter.
- Never eat any combination of beef, lamb and pork more

than three times per week. Choose lean cuts of meat and cut off all visible fat before cooking.

- When preparing chicken or turkey, be sure to cut off the skin before cooking because much of the fat is contained in the skin. Eat the light meat because it contains less fat than the dark meat.
- Eat smaller portions of meat by using dishes that combine meat with vegetables,(especially legumes like beans) pasta or grains.
- Avoid duck, goose, gravies, sauces, casseroles, pot pies, croissants, fried fast foods, prepackaged cake mixes, biscuit mixes, or pancake mixes, ice cream, whole milk, evaporated milk, sweetened, condensed milk, artificial or non-dairy creamers, and bacon bits.

## A little lean meat may not hurt your heart

A diet including lean meat may be "almost as effective" as a vegetarian diet in reducing your risk of heart disease, Australian researchers report in the *American Journal of Clinical Nutrition* (50,2:280).

The real plus is this: more of us would stick to a diet that includes lean meat, the scientists believe.

In the study, 26 men from a fitness center ate one of three different diets — a high-fat "typical Australian" diet, a lean-meat diet, and a milk-egg-vegetable diet — for six-weeks so researchers could compare the risk-reduction benefits.

The diets varied from 2,100 to 3,000 calories per day, based on individual needs as determined by metabolic tests. Only among the milk-egg-vegetable group was there a small loss of weight.

The researchers found that the milk-egg-veggie eaters cut their cholesterol levels by ten percent. The lean-meat eaters cut their total cholesterol by five percent.

Both "healthy" diets had a slight effect on blood pressure, lowering diastolic pressure an average of two to five points.

Participants on the lean-meat diet ate about nine ounces — slightly over a half-pound — of lean meat every day. The lean meat included combinations of processed ham, corned beef, chicken sausage, fresh beef and chicken.

This lean-meat diet replaced 60 percent of the plant protein in the milk-egg-vegetable diet with meat protein.

Incidentally, the high-fat Australian diet was also high in cholesterol and low in fiber — similar to the typical American diet.

Not surprisingly, men on this diet did not do as well as their counterparts on the other two diets.

During the study, researchers checked the participants' heart rate, blood pressure, and serum cholesterol levels every two weeks. They also checked high-density-lipoprotein (HDL or "good") cholesterol and low-density-lipoprotein (LDL or "bad") cholesterol levels.

Although men on the milk-egg-vegetable diet had the greatest reduction in blood pressure and cholesterol levels, the lean-meat diet "did not negate" the lowering of those two risk factors. Men on the high-fat diet had the least reduction, and, thus, the least benefit.

However, the lean-meat diet also reduced "good" cholesterol, although researchers expected the reduction. They say the decline in HDL cholesterol would level off and stabilize over longer periods.

Researchers point out that in the milk-egg-vegetable diet, wheat — not soy — was the principal source of protein. In the current study, eating wheat protein led to an increase in glutamate, an amino acid relative that is linked to an excessive amount of cholesterol in the blood.

Although the lean-meat diet was less effective than the milk-egg-vegetable diet, researchers believe a diet including some lean meat is more acceptable to most people and would stand the best chance of long-term compliance.

# Common Cold

## A better remedy for cold symptoms?

British doctors think they may have come up with a better remedy for the common cold. Their new approach calls for inhaling moist, hot air for 20 minutes, according to the research report in *British Medical Journal* (298,6683:1265). The report says that inhaling humidified air at just under 110 degrees F. shortens the course of the cold and brings many patients next-day relief.

In a controlled study, those who breathed in moist, hot air improved faster than those who inhaled "steamy" air. The warm, steamy air was at about 86 degrees F. Such warm, steamy air can be produced by a common vaporizer. Vaporizers are widely used by cold sufferers to ease their symptoms. However, the air is much hotter than 86 degrees at the exhaust point.

Researchers studied two groups of patients. They found

that the "hot-air" patients did better than the "warm-air" patients. On the fourth day of medical check-ups, 21 of the hot-air patients said their colds were gone.

But only one of the warm-air patients reported no more cold symptoms. However, people in both groups reported their symptoms had been cut nearly in half by the treatments.

In a follow-up study, more volunteers received one 20-minute treatment on the first day and 10-minute treatments each morning after that until their cold symptoms disappeared. The first treatment seemed to benefit them, but the additional treatments didn't seem to do any good, the *BMJ* report says.

"Evidence suggests that 20 minutes of treatment at (110 degrees F.) of an already developed 'natural' cold is beneficial," say the researchers. "Twenty minutes given early in the mild experimental cold gave no continuing benefit, but three treatments at 30 minutes did," the study says. "Treatments of 10 minutes had little effect."

The hotter-air treatment also helped hay fever sufferers, leading researchers to suggest the hot, moist air treatments may have some kind of anti-inflammatory effect.

No bad side effects were reported by any of the patients, the report says. If you try a homemade version of the "warm-air" treatment, be careful not to get burned.

Inhaling unregulated hot air or placing your face near a vaporizer could scald your face, mouth or nasal passages. Trying to "do-it-yourself" could result in painful, possibly dangerous burns.

The people who took part in the experiments did so under careful medical supervision and used specially designed breathing apparatus. So far, we know of no commercially available machine that will deliver moist air at exactly 110 degrees F. safely to your mouth and nose.

But, remember that the experiment showed that even warm, moist air — like that found in a hot shower or a few feet away from a home vaporizer unit — also can produce good results.

# Depression

## A vitamin deficiency may lead to depression

Low levels of the B vitamin, folic acid, have been linked to depression by A. Missagh Ghadirian of McGill University in Montreal says a report in *Psychosomatics*. Dr. Ghadirian found that folic acid supplements relieved depression in people whose depression was caused by low folic acid levels.

Depression, loss of appetite, dizziness, fatigue, and shortness of breath are the first signs of a folic acid deficiency.

Folic acid is a water-soluble vitamin, so extra amounts are usually passed out through the kidneys into the urine within 24 hours. Without regular folic acid, deficiency symptoms may occur after just 100 days of low folic acid intake.

Adults require 400 micrograms of folic acid daily. In addition, pregnant women need 800 micrograms to help prevent birth defects. Nursing mothers should have 500 micrograms each day.

Folic acid is found naturally in yeast, liver, lima beans, whole-grain products, leafy-green vegetables, oranges, asparagus, turnips, peanuts, oats, potatoes, and beans.

Folic acid dissolves in cooking water when foods are heated, so raw foods are a better source of this vitamin.

Many things can interfere with the body's proper absorption of folic acid. Even if you are getting the daily requirement, your body may not be able to use it.

Oral contraceptives, aspirin, acetaminophen (like Tylenol® and Panadol®), Dilantin®, primidone, phenobarbital, methotrexate, pyrimethamine, triamterene, and high doses of vitamin C reduce the amount of folic acid available for the body to use.

The percentage of depressed people who are actually suffering from a folic acid deficiency is not known, the report said.

# Diabetes

## You may be diabetic and not know it

The American Diabetes Association estimates that five million Americans have diabetes and don't know it. Here are the warning signs they list:

- Overweight and over the age of 40
- Excessive thirst
- Easily tired
- Diabetes history in the family
- Change or blurring in vision
- Frequent urination
- Sores heal slowly

If you or anyone you know shows these symptoms, they advise you to get a doctor's help immediately.

# Diabetics die from excess of fat

Diabetics are dying "from an excess of fat," according to the *Journal of the American Medical Association* (262,3:398). Heart and artery disease are the leading causes of death among diabetics.

In addition, research shows that high cholesterol levels are a danger to diabetics. Despite these facts, most diabetics are not aware of their own cholesterol levels.

Even some diabetics who know they have high cholesterol levels are not being treated correctly, a University of Texas study reveals.

More than 40 percent of the people with diabetes had high levels of blood lipids (a cholesterol measurement), compared to similar levels in less than one-fourth of the nondiabetic population, says a study in the *Journal of the American Medical Association* (262,3:360).

Twenty-three percent of the diabetics also had additional risk factors — high triglyceride levels or low levels of HDL (high-density lipoproteins).

The problem is compounded because less than a fourth of the diabetics with cholesterol problems knew that they had problems. What's worse, only 10 percent were receiving treatment, notes Dr. Michael Stern, who led the study.

"We suspect that the low level of awareness and treatment … is probably a general phenomenon," says Stern.

"An excess of fat, an excess of fat in the body (obesity), an excess of fat in the diet, and an excess of fat in the blood" was considered a cause of heart and artery disease in diabetics as early as 1927, an editorial in *JAMA* notes.

"Despite the seven decades that have passed and the considerable knowledge that has been gained since that time, physicians continue to pay little attention to the control of plasma lipid disorders in their diabetic patients," *JAMA* says.

The study by Dr. Stern and an editorial by Dr. George Steiner warn that doctors and diabetic patients must become more aware of the dangers of high cholesterol.

In addition, the articles say, both patient and doctor must learn to treat the dangerous condition through proper diet, weight reduction, or, if necessary, with prescription drugs. "Important though it may be, glycemic (blood sugar) control is not sufficient to provide the best treatment for a diabetic patient," Steiner says.

The American Diabetic Association now recommends that all diabetics have their cholesterol levels checked regularly.

The test should produce a fasting lipid profile, including total cholesterol levels, high-density lipoproteins (HDL), low-density lipoproteins (LDL) and triglycerides.

Each person should keep a personal record of each cholesterol test result to help increase awareness and to provide information in case of an emergency.

If the levels are not within the National Cholesterol Education Guidelines, work with your physician to reach safe levels.

# High-carbohydrate diet may be risky for diabetics

To lower heart-disease risk, the American Heart Association (AHA) recommends a low-fat, high-carbohydrate diet for all Americans. Some researchers contend a high-carbohydrate diet may be harmful for people who are insulin-resistant — namely, diabetics — who cannot process large amounts of carbohydrates, says a report in *Science News* (136,12:185).

Both the AHA and the American Diabetes Association (ADA) recommend that carbohydrates make up 50 to 60 percent of daily caloric intake. Some researchers believe that percentage is too high.

"When patients who have non-insulin-dependent diabetes are given this so-called 'good' diet, they have marked increases in triglycerides [a form of fat in the bloodstream] and a significant decrease in HDL cholesterol [high-density-lipoprotein, or "good" cholesterol]," says diet researcher Ann M. Coulston of Stanford University. "And in patients with diabetes, a rise in triglycerides is associated with an increased risk of cardiovascular disease."

Coulston advocates a diet of 40 to 45 percent total carbohydrates. She and her colleagues conducted a six-week study, giving 12 diabetics two diets for six weeks at a time. Carbohydrates made up 40 percent of total calories in the first diet, and 60 percent in the second (the recommended amount).

"Diabetics on the 60 percent diet had a 30 percent rise in serum triglycerides and a 9 percent decrease in HDL," according to Coulston's report at the ADA meeting last June.

The ADA hasn't been quick to change its dietary guidelines, however. It will wait for further research to confirm these results.

## A way to slow the onset of diabetic blindness

Some degree of vision loss is inevitable for nearly every diabetic, according to Dr. Ronald Klein, ophthalmologist at the University of Wisconsin Medical School. The vision problems facing 11 million American diabetics result from a condition known as diabetic retinopathy. It's the leading cause of new blindness in the U.S. for people between 20 and 75.

But there's new hope for lessening the damage caused by the disease, says a report in *Medical Tribune* (30,20:1). Aspirin and a tight control of blood sugar levels seem to put the brakes on the progress of retinopathy, says Dr. Harold Rifkin, clinical professor of medicine at New York's Albert Einstein College of Medicine. That's especially true in the early stages of the disease.

Researchers in British and French studies found that giving a diabetic an aspirin tablet (330 milligrams) three times daily slowed the deterioration of tiny arteries feeding the eyes. Diabetics also seem to get a good effect by keeping glycemic levels under tight control. Generally, that involves sticking closely to doctor-recommended dietary guidelines.

Severe cases of retinopathy now are treated by laser

flashes that promote clotting of tiny eye hemorrhages. Untreated retinopathy can lead to blindness.

One symptom of the problem is cotton-wool spots — white spots with fuzzy borders — in the field of view. Others include blurred vision and small black spots ("floaters") that move in the field of vision as the eye moves.

Every diabetic patient should get regular eye check-ups from an ophthalmologist who has a special interest in diabetes, recommends Dr. Jeanne L. Rosenthal, attending surgeon at the New York City Eye and Ear Infirmary.

Check with your doctor about the benefits of aspirin for diabetics.

## Pea fiber: good news for diabetics

Danish researchers say the kind of dietary fiber found naturally in peas helps smooth out the usual sharp rise in blood sugar levels right after a meal. That's good news for diabetics, especially, because they sometimes have trouble controlling what's called postprandial (after-meal) glycemia (high levels of blood sugar).

An added bonus: used in regular baked products, the pea fiber tastes okay, too, says the report in the *American Journal of Clinical Nutrition* (50,2:324).

The researchers compared the beneficial effects of a commercial brand of pea fiber available in Denmark to comparable amounts of wheat bran and beet fiber. "The postprandial blood glucose response was markedly reduced by the (pea fiber)," the report says. "Because the palatability is good, it may prove a valuable food additive for diabetics." The wheat bran and beet fiber had almost no effect on either blood glucose or serum insulin levels, the researchers say.

The pea fiber used is a white, almost tasteless granulated powder that is easily baked into bread, the report says. About two-thirds of pea fiber is the water-soluble type. The added pea fiber had no effect on normal bowel movement schedules, the study says.

Only one patient reported any side effects: a feeling of fullness after eating the test meal containing 30 grams (just over one ounce) of pea fiber in a mixture of ground beef and two kinds of sugar.

## A little table sugar may be safe for some diabetics

There may be good news on the horizon for some diabetics. Adding sucrose to their restricted diets had no bad effects on a small group of type-II (non-insulin-dependent) diabetics, according to an Australian study. Sucrose is a natural sweetener that most of us know in its refined form as table sugar.

"Our study suggests that the controlled use of sucrose can be considered in certain [diabetic] individuals," researchers report in the *American Journal of Clinical Nutrition* (50,3:474). The results of this and other studies may redefine the traditional dietary guidelines for diabetics.

Diabetics cannot process natural sugars efficiently. So,

until now, they have been told to avoid table sugar completely. Diabetics regularly use artificial sweeteners such as aspartame, which is why researchers chose it for study.

They studied nine people whose diabetes was well under control. None were taking insulin, and all were in good health. Three were treated with diet only, and six were treated with diet and a drug used to control diabetes.

Researchers randomly assigned participants to one of two groups for six weeks each. One group received one and one-half ounces of sucrose daily, and the second received about five and one-half ounces of aspartame, the amount equivalent in sweetness to sucrose.

The participants did not suffer any harmful effects from the supplements and were able to process sugar effectively, even without the drug.

Total cholesterol, high-density lipoprotein (HDL, or "good") cholesterol and triglycerides (a type of fat in the blood stream) "were not significantly different" at the end of each study period, compared with the levels measured before the study began. The same held true for blood-sugar and insulin levels.

Researchers "caution against overinterpreting the results," emphasizing the following:

- The form of sucrose used is important. Participants used sucrose as an additive, only in coffee or tea or on breakfast cereal. High-fat, high-sugar baked goods were not evaluated.
- Participants must be followed up for long-term side effects.

- Regular "diabetic-type" diet is important. Studies in which sucrose supplemented a high-carbohydrate diet had poor results.
- The study size was small, only nine people. Much larger studies are necessary for more precision in determining accurate results that might apply to most type-II diabetics.

If you are a diabetic, don't try this experiment on your own.

Check with your doctor before making any change in your diet or treatment program.

# Digestive Disorders

## How to help heartburn

"Up to 36 percent of healthy persons report at least one episode of heartburn per month, and 7 percent of these report daily heartburn," according to *Modern Medicine* (57:92).

Repeated attacks of heartburn are known medically as gastroesophageal reflux disease (GERD). GERD is caused when stomach acid "backs up" from the stomach into the esophagus, or food pipe, and causes the familiar discomfort we call heartburn. Actual symptoms can range from a burning sensation to sharp stabs of pain.

Heartburn can be ignited by one or more "triggers," acting alone or in combination with each other. Here are several:

- The lower esophageal sphincter (or LES), a small flap that helps stop acid from backing up. The LES can become relaxed and lose effectiveness.

- Pressure on the stomach.
- Delayed emptying of the stomach.
- Hiatal hernia.
- The content of the material backing up from the stomach.

Since GERD can be a serious medical problem, recurring heartburn should be brought to the attention of your doctor, Dr. John Goff suggests in *Modern Medicine*. Some common GERD symptoms include the following:

- Stomach burning, heartburn, or discomfort.
- Regurgitation for no apparent reason or when you bend over.
- The "sudden filling of the mouth with salty fluid," known as water brash.
- Painful or difficult swallowing.
- Unusual chest pain not associated with the heart.

However, even if GERD is diagnosed, there are many simple steps you can take to help alleviate reflux problems, Goff says.

(1) Raise the head of your bed by six to eight inches. This should create enough difference in the level of your head and your stomach so that the acid cannot flow up out of your stomach.
(2) Do not eat for two to three hours before bedtime. During the day, do not lie down if you are bothered by indigestion. Lying down usually makes the problem worse. Sitting up or standing helps the stomach acids

remain in the stomach.

(3) Avoid caffeine, fat, chocolate and alcohol. Peppermint, aspirin, tea, fried foods, citrus fruits and juices, onion or garlic can also aggravate indigestion and should be avoided or used only in moderation.

(4) If you are taking a prescription drug that is known to aggravate reflux, talk to your doctor about possibly switching to a different drug.

(5) Reduce or eliminate all types of tobacco use.

(6) Lose weight, especially around your waist.

(7) Don't wear tight clothes, girdles or belts.

(8) Reduce the amount of air you swallow by slowing down your eating and avoiding chewing gum.

(9) Suck on lozenges (but not the peppermint-flavored ones). Increasing the flow of saliva by using lozenges can decrease heartburn symptoms.

(10) Avoid the following prescription drugs: theophylline, progesterone, diazepam, Sectral®, Tenormin®, Lopressor®, Corgard®, Visken®, Inderal®, Blocadren®, Timolide®, Cardizem®, Procardia®, Calan®, Isoptin®, Quinidex Extentabs®, phentolamine, Dibenzyline®.

## Is a natural treatment for ulcers on the way?

Years ago, doctors usually had only general advice and one main treatment besides surgery for patients with ulcers.

The advice was "watch what you eat." The customary treatment was "a bland diet," meaning lots of milk, little fiber and no spices.

That's changed considerably in recent years. Doctors now have whole arsenals of drug treatments for ulcer victims. And while doctors still advise us to avoid those foods that irritate the digestive system, bland diets for ulcers seem to have gone the way of cod liver oil.

But the future for ulcer sufferers may contain something of the past. Diet may again take a leading role in managing ulcer disease, according to a report in *FDA Consumer* (23,5:14). During the past two decades, the rates and severity of ulcer attacks have gone down. Many researchers think that's because of changes in our diet, mainly a switch from animal fats and tropical oils in cooking to use of plant protein and vegetable fats.

Many doctors and nutritionists have urged such changes to lower our blood cholesterol levels and reduce our risks of heart disease. The side benefit of that switch may have been fewer ulcers along the way. As a result, researchers are looking into the possibilities of natural ulcer fighters.

Vegetable oils provide polyunsaturated fats, including one essential fatty acid — linoleic acid — that the body requires for processing certain nutrients. Linoleic acid and another polyunsaturated fat, arachidonic acid, help the stomach produce hormone-like substances called prostaglandins. These prostaglandins help protect the stomach's lining and speed up healing.

Researchers hope to learn more about linoleic acid and how it contributes to this natural healing mechanism for ulcers. Your body can make linoleic acid if it's forced to. But nutritionists recommend that you take in about 2 percent of your daily calories in the form of linoleic acid. Good sources include oils made from corn, safflowers and soybeans (but not olive oil or coconut oil).

Even if you are on a strict, low-fat diet, you should take about a tablespoon of such polyunsaturated oil every day, according to *Jane Brody's Nutrition Book* (pg. 56).

Special advice for seniors: sometimes ulcers can strike people over 55 without the usual accompanying symptom of pain. These painless ulcers can stay hidden for a long time and do a lot of damage.

Check with your doctor about your ulcer risk and potential natural ways to manage an ulcer problem.

## Discovered: a revolutionary new way to totally stamp out ulcers

Many ulcers caused by germs? And may even be contagious? That startling suggestion is at the core of what may be a revolutionary new approach to treating ulcer patients.

The treatment — using a pink, over-the-counter antacid and diarrhea fighter — seems to deliver a knockout punch to painful, sometimes life-threatening stomach ulcers.

New research has linked ulcers to a common stomach bacteria. The same study says that the well-known stomach soother, Pepto-Bismol, may play an important role in eliminating both the bacteria and the ulcers.

An Australian researcher first associated ulcers with the Campylobacter pylori bacteria in 1983. Since then, doctors have asked, "Does Campylobacter pylori cause ulcers, or does this bacteria simply show up and thrive where ulcers occur?"

In a recent clinical test, new "triple therapy" — bismuth subsalicylate (Pepto-Bismol) in combination with antibiotics and the ulcer drug ranitidine (brand name Zantac) — eliminated both the bacteria and the internal stomach sores in ulcer sufferers.

This study indicates that healing ulcers and preventing the formation of new ulcers is linked to eliminating the bacteria. Spicy foods and stress levels apparently play much less important roles in ulcer formation than previously thought.

At a recent conference on digestive disorders, Dr. David Graham of the Houston Veterans Administration Medical Center reported that the group taking "triple therapy" only had one ulcer recurrence. But eight of every 10 people in the control group had new ulcers flare up again within six months. Everybody in the control group took only the prescription ulcer drug and nothing else.

"Accelerated healing was observed in the triple therapy group, with nearly twice as many healed at four weeks and 100 percent healed at 12 weeks, compared with 16 weeks needed for total ulcer resolution in the group given only ranitidine," Dr. Graham says in *Medical World News* (30,12:9). Dr. Graham once was vigorously skeptical about a germ-ulcer link. Now he's a believer.

A study by Dr. Thomas Borody, director of the Centre for Digestive Diseases in Sydney, showed that patients who were cleared of Campylobacter pylori remained free of ulcers for 16 months. Take away the bacteria, and — other things being equal — you take away the ulcers, the study indicates. "Duodenal ulcer recurs when Campylobacter pylori recurs," Borody says.

Just how someone "catches" the bacteria is not known. However, when four members of the same family developed ulcers in The Netherlands, doctors found that they all were infected with Campylobacter pylori. So were four other family members living in the same home.

Since all eight people were infected with the identical strain of the bacteria, researchers believe that either they were all infected at the same time or that the bacteria can be transmitted from person to person.

Not all ulcers are associated with the bacteria, according to Dr. Lawrence Laine of the University of Southern California. He says that people with ulcers caused by nonsteroidal anti-inflammatory drugs (NSAIDs) generally aren't infected with the Campylobacter pylori bacteria.

## Blood with bowel movements

One of the more unsettling personal experiences is discovering the presence of blood after a bowel movement. The important question is this: when is blood mixed with bowel movements only a minor irritation, and when is it potentially very serious?

"Rectal bleeding of any degree is always alarming," says *Lancet* (1,8631:195), "with the fear of cancer being uppermost in the patient's mind."

However, the report went on to note that traces of blood on the paper are relatively common and should not be cause for great worry. "A little blood on the paper after defecation is noticed by about one in seven of the adult population," according to the report.

But, "blood in the lavatory pan (toilet bowl) or mixed with the stool (bowel movement), a far more important observation, is seen in only 2 to 3 percent and generally leads to hospital referral," the researchers said.

The general rule of thumb is that if the blood is actually mixed with the bowel movement or is in amounts great enough to stain the water in the toilet bowl, in all cases a doctor should be consulted. But, *Lancet* said, even most of those cases turn out to be more worrisome than dangerous, and most will not require further treatment.

In other words, using the report's statistics, out of 1,000 people, about 142 persons occasionally will notice a little blood on the toilet paper after a bowel movement. Of that 142, only about 20 or 30 persons will have blood mixed with the fecal material itself, an indication of bleeding higher up the anus or intestinal tract and a sign that a doctor's examination is needed.

Of those 30, doctors' examinations and hospital tests will show about nine will have "sizable," non-cancerous polyps (benign tumors) in the bowel or colon. Of those same 30 persons, three will be found to have cancerous growths in the bowel tract, according to the figures given in the *Lancet* report.

# How to put brakes on breaking wind

Benjamin Franklin called it, "Breaking wind." Some say, "Passing gas." The technical term is flatulence, and it has been the source of everything from off-color fraternity jokes for college students to serious attacks of pain — and social embarrassment — for some sufferers.

Almost everybody experiences up to a dozen episodes daily of passing gas. It's the normal by-product of healthy digestion. Unfortunately, in some cases, that gas also can become trapped in folds of the colon and cause mild to severe pain.

"It may feel like a knife stabbing the chest or abdomen," says Dr. John H. Renner. Because the pain can be severe and occurs in areas close to the heart and stomach, many sufferers fear the pain may signal more serious problems like heart disease and ulcers, even cancer.

The gas itself is caused by fermentation, the same process that makes wine. Bacteria are normally present in the digestive tract, according to a report from the American Digestive Disease Society.

When the bacteria work on the undigested parts of a big meal, one by-product is a mixture of gases, including hydrogen sulfide (the familiar rotten egg odor) and smelly residues of fatty acids.

Several things contribute to excess flatulence and gas pain, Renner says. Here are the main ones:

**(1) The kinds of food we eat.** Almost everybody gets gas from eating beans. That's because beans contain two kinds of starches that bacteria love to ferment and that the body can't break down and absorb first. Other problem foods include onions, brussels sprouts, raisins, prune juice, apricots, celery, carrots, bananas, bagels, wheat germ and pretzels, not necessarily in that order.

Sometimes a combination of otherwise innocent foods will trigger excess gas. Keep track of what you eat, compare that with when you experience gas discomfort, and tailor your diet accordingly.

For example, one would not want to eat a large plate of beans or brussels sprouts just before attending a play that contained extended quiet periods. On the other hand, such precautions might not apply before a rock concert.

**(2) Sudden switch to more high-fiber foods.** Most of us need more fiber in our daily diet. But one of the prices we have to pay may be increased flatulence.

"Start with a small dose of fiber so the bowel gets used to it," advises Dr. Michael Mogadam of Georgetown University. "That lessens the increase in flatus." After about two weeks on an increased fiber diet, most people's gas production returns to normal levels.

**(3) Lactase deficiency.** Some people lose the ability to digest milk and milk products efficiently because of a shortage of a digestive enzyme, lactase. Undigested milk sugar gets to the colon and becomes a ripe target for gas-producing bacteria. Try a milk-free diet for two weeks to see if episodes of excess gas decrease. Your doctor can help you zero in on the cause.

**(4) Swallowing air.** Some people actually gulp down large volumes of air while smoking, chewing gum, eating or drinking. Taking smaller bites, chewing them longer, and swallowing smaller amounts of liquid smoothly, without gulping, will help solve that problem.

If chewing gum or smoking are the culprits, abandon the guilty habits. And if you feel like belching, don't help the process, Renner says. Trying to belch just draws in more air, adding to the problem.

**(5) Anxiety.** Being over-anxious or "stressed out" can bring on flatulence. Doctors think stress gives rise to overeating, poor eating habits and impaired digestion processes, all combining to produce excess gas.

When avoiding certain foods or beverages doesn't solve the problem, Renner suggests an over-the-counter product containing simethicone. Simethicone breaks down large gas bubbles trapped in colon folds and may ease painful flare-ups.

The doctor suggests that activated charcoal tablets, available without prescription at most druggists, may also help by absorbing excess gas.

The problem with charcoal is that it also absorbs needed minerals and interferes with many medications. Check with your doctor before using either product.

# Drinking Water

## The truth about 'bottled water'

If you are trying to drink more water every day, you may be among millions of Americans who want something other than what comes out of your home faucet. But, much bottled water may not be any better than water straight from your own tap. In fact, some bottled water comes straight from somebody else's tap.

Bottled water is defined by the U.S. government as "water that is sealed in bottles or other containers and intended for human consumption," according to the *Journal of Nutrition for the Elderly* ((8,1:73).

Read the label carefully to determine which of the following categories the bottled water falls into. Many brands use as part of their brand name the word "spring," but that may have nothing to do with the origin of the water in the bottle.

**Spring water** — If the list of ingredients says spring water, the U.S. Food and Drug Administration requires that the bottled water come from a deep underground source that flows naturally to the surface. Again, forget the brand name. Look at the list of ingredients on the label.

**Natural water** — This must come from a protected underground source. It can be further filtered or purified.

**Drinking water** — This can be just ordinary tap water from a city or county water system that is filtered or treated in some way before bottling. It probably has chlorine in it, and may have other minerals added or deleted during the processing. It can come from a tap, a spring, a well or a lake.

**Club soda** — This is just tap water that has artificial carbonation added to it, as well as mineral salts added for flavoring. It also probably has been filtered.

**Seltzer** — Like club soda, this is artificially carbonated, filtered tap water, except it has no mineral salts added. Usually, it's also salt-free.

**Sparkling water** — May be either naturally or artificially carbonated. Some naturally carbonated water has carbonation added to it during bottling to keep the carbonation level consistent.

**Flavored water** — May be any of the above types with either natural or artificial flavoring added to it, including sugar or sweetening.

**Distilled or demineralized water** — This is water that is processed by distillation or osmotic filtration to remove its mineral and dissolved material content. Usually, this kind of water is not intended for drinking purposes. Distilled water is probably the purest form of water, but drinking it may cause mineral deficiencies if it replaces "hard" water that contains beneficial minerals.

**Mineral water** — The FDA has no regulation for this kind of bottled water. "Since there is no national standard or definition, the term can be misleading," says the journal report. The amounts and kinds of minerals contained in the water can vary greatly from one brand to another and even in the same brand depending on where it's bottled and sold.

The "best" mineral water should contain liberal amounts of beneficial minerals like calcium and magnesium, and low amounts of sodium and heavy metals like lead. The publisher's choice of mineral water brands: Mountain Valley Water from Hot Springs, Ark.

## What you can do about fluoride in your water

Because having fluoride in drinking water is thought by many people to be beneficial, most water filter manufacturers don't buck prevailing wisdom by advertising products that remove fluoride.

Therefore, there are no products available in the U.S. specifically designed to remove fluorine compounds from home tap water, according to Tom Snee, an official of Intec Corp. of Eagan, Minn.

The company makes whole-house units that combine electronic and absorption methods to filter various materials from drinking water.

"There's nothing on the market right now just for fluorine," Snee says.

But, even though manufacturers don't advertise it, activated charcoal units remove some of the fluorides in drinking water, Snee says.

If you want to cut down the level of fluoride in your tap water, a simple activated charcoal filter is about as good as anything currently available, Snee indicates.

By the way, not all fluoride is added to the water at the treatment plant.

Some areas of the country just have more fluoride in the water naturally because of the presence of mineral deposits near rivers, streams and lakes.

# Drug and Food
# Reactions

## New antibiotic blamed for fatal reaction

A 75-year-old man being treated for bronchitis developed severe blood vessel inflammations and hemorrhages and died after taking the new prescription antibiotic known as ofloxacin.

The man was in the hospital being treated for heart failure when he came down with the lung infection. The trouble showed up after he had taken 200 milligrams of ofloxacin twice a day for five days specifically for the bronchitis, according to the report in the *British Medical Journal* (299,6700:685).

He developed a typical drug rash, and numerous blisters and bleeding areas popped up in his mouth and on his hands and feet, the report says. Doctors found blood in his urine and bowel movements. Despite intensive care, he died within two weeks of starting the antibiotic.

Typical reactions from the new fluorinated quinolone drug usually show up as nausea, diarrhea, headache and restlessness, the *BMJ* report says.

"Ofloxacin was probably an important factor in this case," say the attending physicians. "We suggest that because of this, the drug should be used only when other, better-known agents are ineffective."

## Bee stings and beta blockers: a dangerous combination?

A British doctor blames his heart medication for causing a simple wasp sting to endanger his life. The doctor was stung on the head while shifting some logs in his garden, according to his report in *The Lancet* (2,8663:619). Although he had never before experienced an allergic reaction, within 30 seconds itchy patches erupted on his hands and around his waist and hips. Within three minutes, his tongue and lips had swollen, and hives had broken out all over his body.

By the time his wife was able to get him into a car five minutes later and drive him to the hospital, the doctor was going into allergic shock with a dangerous drop in blood pressure. Emergency room doctors gave him hydrocortisone and antihistamines to stop the potentially fatal shock reaction, and he recovered nicely.

The doctor believes the allergic reaction to the wasp sting was greatly aggravated by his prescription heart drug, a beta blocker called atenolol. He had been taking the drug for two years, following a heart attack in 1987.

Beta blockers are a class of heart drugs that acts on the heart to make it reduce the rate and force of its contractions, thus cutting down on the heart's workload. Some beta blockers are being tried in other ways, too, notably to treat some psychiatric illnesses.

"In giving advice — apart from the obvious warnings to avoid bees, wasps, yellow jackets and hornets — doctors might think of mentioning the need for urgent hospital attendance should a person on beta blockers be stung," Dr. D.L. Pedersen writes.

The doctor says he now carries a bee sting kit with appropriate medicine in his golf bag.

## Osteoporosis linked to thyroid medication

A medication commonly prescribed for women—thyroid hormones — poses bone loss dangers for premenopausal women, according to a recent study at the University of Massachusetts Medical School in Worchester. The data showed that such women on long-term therapy with thyroid hormones experienced losses of hip bone mass. They also may face increased risk of hip fractures later in life.

The study of 31 women (all premenopausal) compared their bone densities after five years of thyroid treatment with those of 31 women of similar ages and weights who had not received thyroid hormones. While both groups showed little decrease in lumbar spine densities, the hip bone densities in the thyroid group showed decreases ranging from 10 to 13 percent, as reported in *Science News* (133:359).

They recommended that doctors should more carefully tailor hormone doses to individual needs and monitor thyroid levels diligently.

They said that thyroid doses often are higher than "normal" levels, and such high doses should be given only to "absolutely necessary" cases, such as to women previously treated for thyroid cancer.

## Psoriasis medicine linked to tanning booth death

A 45-year-old woman who was taking a medicine to treat a skin disease died after being burned in a tanning booth, according to an Associated Press report.

Her medicine — psoralen — makes skin more sensitive to light, especially to ultra-violet rays contained in sunshine and concentrated in tanning booths.

The Indiana woman died of burn complications after using a booth in a beauty salon, the news report says. The report says she had been taking the medicine as a treatment for psoriasis, a skin condition that causes scaly and often painful sores.

Used with medically supervised doses of ultra-violet light, psoralen has been a standard psoriasis treatment for several years. It also helps fight a type of skin cancer known as cutaneous T-cell lymphoma. Psoralen is derived from a chemical found naturally in figs, celery, limes and parsley.

The report indicates that people taking psoralen should be very cautious about getting too much exposure to light. Exposure that would be okay for most people may be dangerous for those taking psoralen.

## Blood pressure medication may cause gout

Diuretics are supposed to drain excess sodium from your body, helping to keep high blood pressure under control. Because they flush the kidneys so effectively, they are known by many people as water pills.

But there are increased reports of elderly women suffering from attacks of gout, a sudden flare-up of pain in their hands or knees, apparently triggered by the diuretics.

"We are finding this in a population over the age of 70, as opposed to the usual gout sufferer, who is usually about 40," says Dr. Steven R. Weiner in *The Western Journal of Medicine* (150,4:419). "We are seeing women more commonly than men, which is a total reverse," says Weiner.

If you are taking water pills, you may be susceptible to this drug reaction, indicates the report. Even if you have osteoarthritis, suspect diuretic-caused gout if your hand suddenly becomes very painful in the joints and shows evidence of inflammation, suggests Weiner.

If this happens, don't try to treat yourself or to change your medication on your own. Check with your regular doctor about what needs to be done.

## 'Water pills' may disrupt heart rhythms

If you take thiazide diuretics — "water pills" — to control your mild or moderate high blood pressure, your heart may be starving for two vital minerals, warns a report in *American Family Physician* (40,5:256).

Long-term use of thiazide medicines may drain potassium and magnesium along with the excess water from your tissues, the report says.

Shortages of those two nutrients can cause the heart to misfire, resulting in increased numbers of what's known as ventricular premature complexes.

When that happens, the heart muscle quivers between beats — something called arrhythmias.

The misfires increase with exercise, the report says.

Bad heart rhythms make the heart beat less efficiently, overworking a muscle already strained by high blood pressure.

A string of such bad rhythms could completely disrupt the normal beating, in effect, stopping the heart. That's what happens to victims of electrical shock — the jolt of current knocks the heart's normal electrical pulses out of kilter.

Doctors often prescribe potassium supplements for their patients taking thiazide medicines.

But they just as often neglect to recommend more magnesium, the report says.

"In addition to potassium supplementation, magnesium supplementation should also be considered in patients who receive thiazide diuretics," the report warns. Check with your doctor before taking or changing medicines.

## Diuretic drug plus dieting can be fatal

A woman lost 22 pounds and her life, probably because she combined a popular low-protein diet with diuretic drugs to lose weight, all without her doctor's knowledge, says a report in *The Lancet* (2,8662:572). The 59-year-old woman was found dead in bed seven weeks after going on the "Cambridge diet," says Dr. C.E. Connolly.

She had lost about 22 pounds, down to 185, during the six weeks she stayed on the low-protein diet. She skipped a week, and died a day after resuming the diet, the report says.

"She had complained of headache and dizziness for a few days before her death, but did not go to see her doctor," according to the report.

Officials discovered the woman had been taking diuretics on and off for several years. She apparently was under the impression that the "water pills" would help her lose weight. She probably died when her heart rhythms went haywire, the doctor says.

Several people on low-protein diets have died in recent years. Drastic, "crash" dieting and too much of a diuretic can cause big disruptions in the body's normal electrolyte balance. Low-protein diets can starve the heart muscle itself, Dr. Connolly says. Both problems can lead to jumbled heart rhythms and death.

Makers of the Cambridge diet products warn in literature sent to doctors that diuretics should be avoided while on the diet, the report says.

Lessons to be learned: don't go on a crash diet without checking with your doctor. And don't "self-medicate" with drugs that may have dangerous side effects and interactions with other drugs or food.

## Serious side effects of some arthritis drugs

Heavy doses of several common arthritis drugs can cause severe side effects, especially in those over age 50, a medical report warns.

The side effects include ulcers, stomach bleeding, ringing in the ears, lightheadedness, slurred speech, difficulty with concentration, confusion, memory loss, hallucinations, paralysis and even death, according to *Geriatrics* (44,4: 95).

People with arthritis who need to take high doses of these drugs over many months or years are at highest risk of suffering from these dangerous side effects, the medical journal says.

The elderly are at an increased risk because their liver and kidneys do not work as well. When kidneys get sluggish with age, the body doesn't clear out the drugs as quickly, leading to more serious side effects than experienced by younger people.

Elderly people often take many different drugs and make mistakes in taking their medicine, which further increases their risk of side effects, notes the researcher writing in *Geriatrics*.

As a group, the elderly are seven times more likely than the general population to experience adverse drug reactions," the report says.

Studies show that up to four percent of patients on continuous therapy with certain arthritis drugs, known as NSAIDs, may have serious gastrointestinal reactions, like peptic ulcers and stomach bleeding. These dangerous side effects can occur without warning symptoms and can lead to death.

NSAIDs are non-steroidal anti-inflammatory drugs, including aspirin and ibuprofen. They are used to treat arthritis, menstrual cramps and general pain.

"Current users of prescription NSAIDs were over four times more likely to die from peptic ulcer or upper gastrointestinal hemorrhage than non-users," reports Marie R. Griffen in the *Annals of Internal Medicine* (109:359).

Since "the non-aspirin NSAIDs are among the most widely prescribed drugs ... even relatively small risks may have major public health implications," Griffen says.

According to the FDA, studies indicate that one out of 100 patients treated for three to six months suffers some of these serious effects at some time during the treatment. For every 100 patients treated with NSAIDs for one year, two to four will experience ulcers and stomach bleeding.

Memory loss, difficulty with concentration, irritability,

lightheadedness, disorientation and exhaustion have also been linked to NSAIDs, *Geriatrics* reports.

Gold compounds may cause severe central nervous system problems like delirium, cranial nerve palsy, tremor, pain syndrome and paralysis.

In addition, large doses of aspirin can lead to hearing loss or ringing in the ears, called tinnitus.

Usually these hearing problems are reversible, and just stopping the aspirin treatment or reducing the dose can help reduce the side effects.

If you notice any of these side effects, contact your doctor immediately. Many times the dose or drug can be changed, and the side effect eliminated.

However, don't stop taking or change the dose of any drug without consulting your doctor first.

# Heart drugs that may be dangerous

Two prescription heart-rhythm drugs have been associated with an increased rate of heart attacks and deaths and were recently withdrawn from a five-year study by the National Institutes of Health (NIH).

According to *Science News* (135,17:260), patients in the study who took encainide (brand name Enkaid) and flecainide (brand name Tambocar) "showed a two- to three-fold greater risk of cardiac arrest or death compared with patients taking placebo after an average treatment period of 10 months." (A placebo is a harmless, ineffective "medicine" given to a group of patients as a control to test the effectiveness of a genuine drug given to another group of patients.)

Enkaid and Tambocor have been prescribed for several years by physicians for patients with severe cases of irregular heartbeat.

The two drugs are used to regulate the heartbeat rate. Bristol Laboratories, manufacturer of Enkaid, and 3M Riker, maker of Tambocor, estimate that 200,000 Americans currently take these drugs.

However, because of the study results, the Food and Drug Administration (FDA) is now warning doctors and other health professionals that use of Enkaid and Tambocor should be limited to use by patients with irregular heartbeats that are "immediately life-threatening."

Otherwise, the two drugs should be used only in very rare cases when people have less-threatening heart rhythm irregularities, according to the report of the FDA warning.

The drugs were withdrawn from the Cardiac Arrhythmia Suppression Trial when an independent safety monitoring board discovered the high death rate.

Fifty-six of 730 patients given one of these two drugs had died from some cause or suffered a heart attack, compared with 22 deaths out of 730 patients given the harmless placebo. "Specifically, 33 taking one of the two drugs experienced sudden cardiac death or a nonfatal heart attack, compared with 9 in the placebo group," *Science News* said.

People taking these drugs should *not* stop taking them, but should discuss this with their doctors, say the FDA and NIH researchers.

# Common over-the-counter painkiller linked to serious kidney damage

Long-term use of acetaminophen, a widely used painkiller, has been linked to kidney damage, according to researchers in North Carolina.

Acetaminophen is the main painkilling ingredient in such over-the-counter medications as Tylenol, Datril, Panadol and Anacin-3.

"We found an increased risk associated with daily use of acetaminophen," says the study in the *New England Journal of Medicine* (320,19:1238).

The researchers compared the effects on the kidneys of long-term use of acetaminophen, aspirin and another kind of painkiller called phenacetin.

Kidney damage was linked to regular use of acetaminophen and phenacetin, but not to aspirin.

Since 1983, "phenacetin has been removed from most combination analgesics (painkillers) because of reported association with chronic renal (kidney) disease and urologic (bladder) cancers, and acetaminophen has replaced phenacetin in many popular combination analgesics (painkillers)," the study reports.

"Regular use of acetaminophen-aspirin combinations, especially when taken jointly with caffeine," was also strongly associated with kidney damage, says a *New England Journal of Medicine* editorial (320,19:1269).

"The 1989 *Physicians' Desk Reference* lists more than 75

combinations of aspirin, acetaminophen, and caffeine, in addition to many preparations that contain only one ingredient," the editorial says.

Because of the many products containing acetaminophen and the potential dangers, the National Institutes of Health (NIH) consensus conference suggested that "sales of analgesics over the counter be limited to preparations containing a single agent."

"The risk increased with the number of pills taken each day by daily users and the frequency of use, but the odds ratios did not increase with years of use after five years," says head researcher Dale P. Sandler.

In addition, there was another danger. Caffeine taken with the painkiller also increased the kidney damage risk. Caffeine is a standard ingredient in many such preparations.

Kidney disease caused by painkillers can be severe and can lead to the need for dialysis or a kidney transplant.

Thirteen percent of people needing dialysis in Australia and 16.8 percent of patients requiring dialysis or transplants in West Germany suffered the kidney damage as a direct result of long-term use of painkillers, the report says.

"Acetaminophen has been available in the United States without a prescription since 1955, but aspirin substitutes did not become popular until the early 1970s," says the study.

A 1980 survey found that acetaminophen accounted for almost one-fourth of all sales of painkillers.

Other painkillers, like ibuprofen, have also been linked to kidney damage. Ibuprofen, available over-the-counter as Advil, Nuprin, Medipren and other brands, is a nonsteroidal anti-inflammatory drug

It is also known to cause kidney problems with long-term use. However, ibuprofen was not among the painkillers included in this study.

Many cold, allergy and sinus medications also include acetaminophen as one of the active ingredients. Be sure to read the ingredients listed on the label or box of a product before buying it.

# Eye Problems

## Fatigued? It may be your eyes

With the fast-paced life of many Americans, many people seem to be suffering from more fatigue. But the reason for the tiredness may be directly related to one's eyesight. People should make sure they are getting adequate sleep, daily exercise, and a well-balanced diet before considering other causes of fatigue. However, many doctors warn that the eye may be the key to unusual tiredness.

Old prescription glasses, improper contact lenses, or deteriorating eyesight can cause extreme fatigue, doctors warn. If you are tired, get an eye exam. Using glasses or contacts that are not strong enough for your needs can put great strain on your eyes and zap your energy. An eye exam may uncover a visual problem that has been causing your tiredness.

People with high blood pressure, diabetes, or a history of vision problems should have an eye exam by an ophthalmologist once a year. Everyone should see an eye doctor at least once every two years, according to the National Society to Prevent Blindness.

For elderly persons on modest budgets or fixed incomes, a helping hand for eye treatment is available. The Eye Care Project Helpline is a toll-free number sponsored by the Foundation of the American Academy of Opthalmology. Call 1-800-222-EYES if you are over age 65 and have limited financial means. An advisor will refer you to a participating local eye doctor who will charge no more than Medicare or insurance limits for eye examination and treatment.

Wearing the "correct" sunglasses can cut certain aging processes in your eyes by up to six-fold, according to a report from Research to Prevent Blindness (RPB), a leading voluntary organization in support of eye research. "Correct" means lenses that block out a high percentage (at least 90 percent) of the harmful ultraviolet (UV) light present in natural sunlight, and frames that position the lenses so that little sunlight seepage occurs around the edges and over the top. UV is light at the shortwave end of the color spectrum and is responsible for sun-tanning, among other effects.

UV light "appears to accelerate aging of receptors of human vision, and cumulative exposure speeds up aging of the lens of the eye, contributes to cataract formation and possible changes in the retina (the screen of the eye), leading to macular degeneration," said Dr. John S. Werner, professor of psychology and neurosciences at the University of Colorado. Macular degeneration, the impairment of the central area of the retina, is the major cause of blindness in those over age 60.

You can test yourself for signs of macular degeneration,

according to *Your Good Health*, a 1987 Harvard University publication. Look at a page of print; if the fine detail in the center seems blurred while the edges seem okay, you need to check with an opthalmologist. Another test is this: see if the lines on a sheet of graph paper appear broken or distorted where you are looking, but not near the edges. If distortion appears, see your doctor.

Normally, the eye's natural lens filters out much of the UV we get in sunlight, even on cloudy days. If the natural lens is removed — for cataract surgery, for example — the UV rays speed through to hit and damage the retina, the main vision area of the eye. Dr. Werner and associates studied eight patients who had cataractous lenses removed from both eyes and then had plastic lenses implanted. On each patient, one eye was implanted with a plastic that absorbed 90 percent of the UV hitting it, while the other eye got a plastic lens that filtered out only 14 percent.

Five years later, while both eyes appeared superficially healthy, on the eye that received more UV, "our psychophysical tests showed loss in the shortwave cone sensitivity from chronic exposure to UV (radiation)," Dr. Werner reported to a RPB seminar on new findings about UV hazards. "Five years of chronic exposure to UVR produced an average loss in shortwave cone sensitivity equal to about 30 years of normal aging."

While UV damage to the eyes is long-term and cumulative, experts are now warning all who spend any time outdoors to wear properly fitting sunglasses to avoid further bad effects. "You can't ignore the hazard in any season or location," Dr. Werner said.

Good UV-shielding sunglasses don't have to be expensive, according to *American Journal of Public Health* (78,1:72). Researchers tested 32 pairs of sunglasses, each costing less than $7, and found that most of them filtered out 98 percent or more of the harmful UV rays in sunlight. Glass and plastic lenses were equally effective in blocking UV, the study showed.

The problem was in the fit of the glasses on the head, particularly in whether the glasses allowed some sunlight (and UV) to "seep" around the edges of the lenses into the eyes. Using a mannequin and light detectors in place of eyes, researchers discovered that UV leaked around the tops and sides of the frames. They also found that wearing the sunglasses even a third of an inch down the nose increased UV penetration by as much as 45 percent.

The lesson is this: check the labels to make sure the sunglasses will block out almost all UV (check with the merchant to be sure), and buy large-framed glasses contoured to your face to block out UV seepage from the sides and top. And wear them as close to your eyes as possible.

At the same time, be aware of the "sunglasses syndrome," as reported by three Harvard Medical School doctors in the publication *Your Good Health*. Sunglasses syndrome signals include numbness and unpleasant sensations beneath the eyes, inside the nose, over the cheeks, and eventually around the upper front teeth and gumline.

Such symptoms may indicate that your sunglasses, if large and heavy, are compressing a sensory nerve. That nerve emerges from the bone about a half inch away from the nose and a little under each eye. Heavy sunglasses, worn for long periods, may pinch that nerve, producing numb gums and other uncomfortable sensations in the facial area. Get relief by removing the glasses. Padding also may help.

# The danger of soft contact lenses

Nearly 13 million Americans enjoy the convenience of soft contact lenses, but physicians warn that long-term wear and poor hygiene may lead to a number of eye diseases and illnesses. The warning is especially important for the five million people who use extended-wear lenses.

A special report on ocular diseases in *Postgraduate Medicine* (86,4:90) recently outlined contact-lens injuries and ways you can prevent eye injuries.

• **Conjunctivitis.** Conjunctivitis, the most common eye disease, is inflammation of the mucous membrane lining the eyelid and part of the eyeball. It results from poor hygiene and affects ten percent of soft contact lens wearers each year

There are many types of conjunctivitis, but generally, symptoms include irritation, itching, puffiness, burning and mucous discharge. You may have the sensation of a foreign body in the eye and may awake with swollen eyelids and matted eyelashes. The infection may start in one eye and quickly move to the other.

Proper hygiene will prevent conjunctivitis. Your eye doctor will probably remind you of the importance of soaking lenses in enzymatic solution every week to kill bacteria.

• **Corneal abrasions.** Abrasions or scratches usually occur when inserting or removing lenses. Symptoms include irritation, redness, pain and tearing.

Physicians prescribe antibiotic drops or ointment to use for four or five days until symptoms disappear.

• **Corneal ulcers.** "Trauma, underlying [eye] disease, and contact lens use are the three principal causes of bacterial corneal ulcers," which may cause permanent scarring and blindness if an ulcer erupts. Seven thousand people suffer corneal ulcers each year, and the number will increase as more people try extended-wear lenses.

The disease comes on quickly. Symptoms include pain, discharge, diminished vision, eyelid swelling and sensitivity to light. Physicians treat corneal ulcers with topical antibiotics (a cream or ointment) until the infection clears up. Some patients need hospitalization for further antibiotic treatment, and corneal transplants may be necessary if scarring is permanent.

• **Keratitis.** Keratitis is another form of corneal ulcer, caused by resistant bacteria that contaminate homemade saline solutions and contact lens cases. People who wear soft contact lenses overnight are ten to fifteen times more likely to get keratitis than daily wearers. Long-term wear cuts off the eye's oxygen supply, causing cells on the surface to die and form an ulcer, which may become infected, says a report in *Science News* (136,13:197).

Keratitis is becoming more common because the use of

extended-wear lenses is increasing. Symptoms include pain, sensitivity to light, and some loss of vision. Often, patients do not respond to early treatment. Keratitis is difficult to treat because the bacteria can transform itself into antibiotic-resistant forms. Corneal transplants are often necessary, and even after transplantation, the infection may recur.

If you have any of the symptoms described above, remove your lenses and see your eye doctor.

---

## Tips on preventing contact-lens injury

- Practice good hygiene. Wash your hands before inserting your lenses, and use sterile, commercially prepared saline solution. Follow disinfection guidelines, and *never use homemade preparations*. If you have extended-wear lenses, remove them at least every seven days for cleaning. (Some physicians recommend cleaning extended-wear lenses every day.)

- Don't wear your lenses overnight.

- If your eyes are irritated, don't wear your lenses.

- If you have pain, eyelid swelling or a discharge, see your eye doctor.

# Common household products can cause severe eye injury

If liquid automatic dishwashing detergent splashes in your eyes, get to a doctor quickly, according to a report in *Emergency Medicine* (21,15:53).

Granular dishwashing detergents scratch and irritate the cornea, a transparent coating over the iris and pupil, and may cause serious injury.

Dr. Edward P. Krenzelok, director of the Pittsburgh Poison Center at Children's Hospital in Pittsburgh, "analyzed all cases of exposure to liquid automatic dishwashing detergent reported to the Pittsburgh Poison Center over a 15-month period." Twenty-three cases involved the eyes, and the injuries were more serious than skin exposures or ingestions.

"More than 90 percent of the ocular exposures resulted in symptoms," according to the report. "The irritations were minor corneal abrasions in 74 percent of the cases, but four adults had more extensive corneal abrasions."

In addition, getting shampoo in your eyes may mean more than just momentary stinging. A particular detergent contained in many shampoos could also cause damage to the cornea.

The detergent, sodium lauryl sulfate (SLS), is a common ingredient in soaps and shampoos, and even a drop of SLS is absorbed quickly by the cornea, according to Dr. Keith Green, professor of opthalmology at the Medical College of Georgia.

The chemical accumulates in the clear tissue and stays there for up to five or six days, Dr. Green said in a report to

Research to Prevent Blindness, a leading voluntary organization devoted to eye research and vision protection.

The absorbed SLS, Dr. Green said, causes changes in the amounts of some proteins in the eye, and creates a new kind of protein, not yet identified, in the eyes of rabbits treated in experiments. This raises questions about long-term effects on the normally clear cornea, Dr. Green warned.

A further danger is that SLS in the eye delayed healing of the corneal epithelium — the cellular surface of the clear tissue. Tissue that would have healed in two days instead took ten, Dr. Green said.

While there are no signs of damage to the eye from SLS immediately after shampoo use, far more subtle effects may show up over a long period, Dr. Green warned.

"Our findings lead us to call for more judicious use of detergents such as SLS by both manufacturers and users of soaps and shampoos," Dr. Green reported. "This is particularly true when possible accidental exposure to SLS could occur in infants, where growth is occurring, and in any instance where a healing process is taking place."

The eyes of very young persons and those in a healing stage are most susceptible to SLS damage, the report said. For adults, especially in middle and later years, SLS is suspected to be a factor in causing cataracts, Dr. Green said.

Not all shampoos or soaps contain SLS, so read the labels on such products, and use those without the suspect ingredient, Dr. Green advised.

# Prevent cataracts naturally

People who take regular daily doses of either vitamin C or vitamin E may slash by more than half their risk of developing blinding cataracts, a new scientific study suggests. Those results come from a Canadian study of 175 cataract patients and 175 people without cataracts, according to a report in *Science News* (135,20:308). All those studied were over age 55.

"The scientists found that the only significant difference between the two groups, other than the presence of cataracts, was that the cataract-free individuals had taken at least 400 international units (one regular capsule) of vitamin E and/or a minimum of 300 milligrams of vitamin C per day over the last five years," the report says.

Most of the cataract-free people took only one of the two vitamins in the form of supplements. Those who took extra vitamin C showed a risk reduction of 70 percent, the report says. Those who took vitamin E supplements had a 50 percent reduction in cataract risk.

This study backs up other recent research that also shows dramatic blindness prevention benefits for people using these two vitamins. One doctor, Charles Kelman, recommends taking 1000 to 2000 milligrams (one to two grams) of vitamin C (ascorbic acid) daily to help prevent cataracts. Scientists don't know for sure why the vitamins prevent cloudy formations in aging eyes. Those clouds across the field of vision are caused by proteins being oxidized in the lens of the eye and then clumping together. Some researchers believe that vitamins C and E, both of which are anti-oxidants, neutralize the lens proteins before they can clump together.

Two out of every 10 people between the ages of 60 and 75 in the United States have cataracts. The condition, which can lead to blindness, accounts for a half million surgical operations every year.

"If you could delay cataract formation by just ten years you would eliminate the need for half of the cataract extractions," according to Allen Taylor, who works for the USDA Human Nutrition Research Center on Aging in Medford, Mass.

Cataracts may be caused or triggered by several things, including sunlight (ultra-violet rays), diabetes, steroids and X-rays.

However, vitamins C and E aren't the only powerful natural cataract fighters available. Beta-carotene and riboflavin (vitamin B2) also may help prevent the eye-clouding growths. People with higher than average intakes of vitamin C, vitamin E and beta-carotene (known as antioxidant vitamins) "are at a reduced risk of cataract development," according to H. Gerster in a German study (*Z Ernahrungswiss* 28,1:56).

Other studies by P. Jacques confirm that people with "high levels of at least two of the three vitamins (C, E and B2)" are at reduced risk of developing cataracts compared to people with low levels of these vitamins, reports *Archives of Ophthalmology* (106,3:337).

Harold Skalka has found that a deficiency of riboflavin (vitamin B2) can lead to cataract development, especially in older adults. "Older cataract patients had more riboflavin deficiency. An absence of riboflavin deficiency was found in our older patients with clear lenses," Skalka reports in the *American Journal of Clinical Nutrition* (34,5:861).

In earlier studies reported in *Lancet* (8054:12-3), Skalka suggested that cataracts "may be corrected by dietary restrictions or supplements" of riboflavin. However, "large doses of niacin (vitamin B3) may ... increase the chances of getting cataracts," according to *Vitamin Side Effects Revealed* (FC&A Publishing).

## Unseen bathroom visitors may endanger your eyesight

Your bathroom may be the vacation home of vision-threatening pseudomonas germs. If you wear contact lenses, you may be doubly at risk.

"Pseudomonas love warm, moist environments," says Dr. Louis Wilson, professor of ophthalmology at Emory University in Atlanta, Ga. "Aside from their natural habitat in soil, grass and foliage, the bathroom is probably this bacteria's idea of heaven."

The germs are brought in from the outside in a variety of ways, usually on shoes or clothing. They thrive in and around the bathroom lavatory, the shower and the toilet. A good germ breeding area is in the gooey underside of soap bars in the soap holders of the shower and lavatory. Unfortunately, the bathroom is also where most people put in and take out their contact lenses.

"People get pseudomonas on their hands, then contaminate their (contact lens) solutions," Dr. Wilson says.

The germs grow quickly in homemade saline solutions, the liquid soaking mixtures made by dissolving salt tablets in distilled water, the doctor says. That's because the sterile distilled water may become contaminated with germs once it's opened and other things added to it.

Wilson says the bacteria can also grow well in large containers of a store-bought solution. The germs get in when the contact lens wearer frequently opens, closes and pours the solution, offering many chances for contamination.

Another germ risk happens when you pour the soaking solution from a large bottle into a travel-sized bottle that may have been used for other purposes earlier and may contain germs.

Even with all the chances for bacteria to get into your eyes, you probably are pretty safe unless you scratch the surface of your eye. That scratch provides an opening for the germs to get in and cause an infection. And, unfortunately, contact lens wearers are more likely to get eye scratches than people who don't use contacts, Dr. Wilson warns.

The danger arises when a germ-contaminated lens is put into an eye that has a scratch. Pseudomonas grow quickly, and within 12 hours, the eye will be painful. By the 24-hour mark, the infected eye will have reached the "big trouble" stage, according to Dr. Wilson.

Left untreated, loss of vision and even loss of the eye itself is possible after 36 to 48 hours, Dr. Wilson said.

Symptoms of serious infections requiring immediate medical care include redness, sensitivity to light, and a pain that becomes an ache.

"If you think you have an eye infection, see an ophthalmologist immediately," Dr. Wilson says.

Preventive measures include careful handling of contact lens solutions and use of only medically sterilized containers. Buying solutions in bulk may not be wise, especially if you open and close the bulk container a lot. Better to use smaller, sterile containers, and steer clear of homemade solutions.

An expensive alternative is the new, disposable contact lenses. Wear them a week, then throw them away.

Even if you don't wear contact lenses, be careful about rubbing your eyes with unwashed hands, especially if you may have scratches on the eye surface. And since germs multiply in the gooey part underneath the soap bar, use a platform on the soap dish to keep the bar dry, and wash off the bar first in hot water before washing your hands.

## Migraines may cause vision loss

One of every three migraine-headache sufferers loses her peripheral vision, according to a new study in *Ophthalmology*.

Peripheral vision is "corner of your eye" sight. In other words, if you focus on an object straight ahead, you can still see things in a wide arc off to the sides.

Elderly people are at the highest risk for losing this ability, the report says.

Ten to 12 million Americans suffer from migraines, and they are three times more common among women than men.

Researchers are studying why migraines cause the loss of peripheral vision.

# Fitness and Exercise

## Aerobic exercise and heart disease

Exercise speeds up the removal of triglycerides, a common form of fat, from the bloodstream and reduces the risk of heart disease, according to new research from Rockefeller University. Carefully controlled workouts reduced the fasting blood levels of triglycerides by 16 percent. Exercise also reduced levels of triglyceride-rich lipoprotein by 32 percent after a fat-containing meal, the researchers report.

These fatty particles, which flood the bloodstream after a meal, may deposit part of their unneeded fatty load onto the walls of arteries. Such dumping of fat onto the artery walls could set the stage for a heart attack, the scientists say in a report in *Circulation* (79,5: 1007).

The workouts in the study involved 29 half-hour sessions of jogging on a treadmill over a period of seven weeks. The men in the study jogged an average of 15 miles per week.

"Based on our results, we think the primary effect of exercise training on lipoprotein metabolism is to increase clearance of triglyceride-rich particles from the blood," says Dr. Jan L. Breslow, head of the university's biochemical genetics and metabolism laboratory. "This may be one mechanism whereby exercise might reduce the risk of coronary heart disease."

The investigators noticed that exercise caused a significant increase in activity of an enzyme, lipoprotein lipase. This enzyme breaks down the triglyceride in the dietary fat particles.

In addition, a test to evaluate the men's physical fitness showed their maximum oxygen consumption increased 43 percent as a result of the exercise program. The test results showed that the men developed better fitness at the same time they decreased their blood-fat levels, the scientists say.

This is the first study that separates the effects of exercise from those of diet change and weight loss, which can also reduce blood levels of triglycerides, says Breslow. "During the exercise phase of the study, we increased the calories in their diet slightly so they wouldn't lose weight."

Weight loss is well-known as a means of lowering lipoprotein levels, the researchers note, so "from a clinical view, the great benefit (to patients) would be to combine exercise and weight loss."

Doctors have known for years that exercise helps prevent heart disease. But until this study, scientists didn't know exactly how exercise helps to do that.

# Fitness a key to lower stroke risk

"One way to reduce your risk of joining the half million Americans each year who suffer a stroke is to stay physically fit," says a report in *The Physician and Sportsmedicine* (17,9:37).

Researchers at the Dallas-based Institute for Aerobics Research studied the rates of stroke among 8,421 initially healthy people for an eight-year period. They found that of those otherwise healthy people, the ones who were classified as "high fit" were almost three times less likely to suffer a stroke as those in the "low fit" category. They assigned the people to either high, low or medium fitness levels based on treadmill tests.

This is the first large study to suggest any link between fitness levels and risks of non-fatal stroke, the report says. This "preliminary" finding doesn't surprise Dr. Joseph C. Maroon, director of neurosurgery at a Pittsburg hospital. He notes that fit people usually have high levels of HDL ("good") cholesterol in their bloodstreams. That helps carry off the type of cholesterol that clogs blood vessels.

Several studies suggest that exercise lowers the risk of artery blockages. Artery blockage is pretty much the same thing, whether in the heart or in the brain, he reasons. And artery blockages lead to tissue death, whether brain cells or heart muscle, Maroon says. Because of that, he sees exercise as beneficial for potential stroke victims as well as for people with heart attack risks.

# No age limit on exercise benefits

Even elderly people who are frail can improve their overall health and mobility with appropriate exercises, says a researcher at the University of Michigan School of Medicine. Such exercises may even keep some aged people out of nursing homes, says Tom Hickey, one of the researchers.

Seventy-five patients ranging in age from 65 to 98 tried a simple exercise program for six weeks.

They tried "gentle neck and shoulder rolls, spinal twists, side stretches, feet and arm extensions, flexes and circles, and slow, deep breathing," according to the report in *Geriatrics* (44,6:13).

"Most of the patients were overweight and never exercised regularly," says the report. In addition, many of them suffered from arthritis, high blood pressure, diabetes, heart disease or a combination of the diseases.

They exercised twice a week in the program called SMILE, which stands for So Much Improvement with Little Exercise.

After six weeks, most of them reported less stiffness in the joints and said they had more energy. The researchers noted some drops in high blood pressure readings and in the times required to walk a certain distance.

"Regular exercise may prolong independent living and help keep frail older persons out of nursing homes," the researchers say.

# Moderate exercise helps you live longer

Calling all couch potatoes!

The results are in: regular exercise could help you fight off heart attack and live longer.

A study in the *Journal of the American Medical Association* (262,17:2395) shows that moderate, regular exercise decreases heart-attack risk by as much as 20 percent in middle-aged men.

Women benefit as well, researchers say.

Regular exercisers also are less likely to suffer from stroke, high blood pressure and some forms of cancer, the study says.

Researchers followed 10,224 men and 3,120 women for an average of eight years. Before the study began, everyone was tested on a treadmill and then assigned to a fitness category.

None of the participants had ever had a stroke, diabetes, heart attack or high blood pressure—conditions that would have influenced the results.

During the study, 283 (240 men, 43 women) participants died.

Among men, the primary causes of death were heart disease and cancer.

Among women, cancer was the biggest killer, followed by "other illnesses." Heart disease ranked third.

An editorial accompanying the *JAMA* report points out that time-saving technology has decreased our activity levels, especially at home.

Do you use the remote control to change TV channels rather than get off the sofa to change them yourself? Use a riding lawn mower? An electric snow blower? Electric garage door opener?

Conveniences such as these are turning Americans into couch potatoes.

But here's the good news: couch potatoes — people who don't exercise at all — benefit the most after starting an exercise program, according to the report.

Physically fit people also benefit from increased exercise, but the benefits are not as great.

You don't have to run marathons to get in shape. You can walk your way to physical fitness.

In fact, a brisk, 30-minute walk each day is ideal because walking is fun, easy to do and requires no special equipment. You also can walk at your own pace.

But you must make exercise part of your daily routine, researchers said.

Of course, you should talk to your doctor before starting an exercise program, especially if you have health problems.

Moderate exercise will increase your ability to reason and remember. And those abilities increase as activity levels increase, according to a report in *Psychology and Aging* (4,2:183).

"If people want to maintain mental abilities as they get older, they should exercise on a regular basis," says Dr. Louise Clarkson-Smith, an author of the report.

# Keep your brain young — walk!

Routine, easy aerobic exercise like walking may help the brain perform better as we get older, according to a new study at the University of Southern California.

In tests in animals, Dr. Mohamed A. Fahim found low levels of neurotransmitters in inactive animals and higher levels in animals that had exercised regularly.

Neurotransmitters help the brain communicate with muscles. With good communication and adequate levels of neurotransmitters, your brain can control your muscles. But uncoordination and other signs of advanced aging will occur with low levels, Fahim discovered.

However, all is not lost if you have been leading an inactive life.

Regular aerobic exercise can help restore the levels of neurotransmitters in about five months, Fahim concluded.

Aerobic exercise doesn't necessarily mean exhaustive workouts in a gym.

Walking is one of the best overall aerobic exercises and is recommended for people of all ages. Just walking for 20 minutes, three times a week, will provide excellent aerobic activity.

Be sure to check with your doctor before starting a new exercise program.

# Arthritis patients said to benefit from moderate aerobic exercise

Aerobic exercise can actually decrease joint pain while improving muscle strength and aerobic capacity in people with arthritis, according to a new report in *The Physician and Sportsmedicine* journal (17,2:128).

It has always been difficult for arthritis patients and doctors to balance the need for exercise with the joints' need for rest.

However, three doctors at the University of Michigan say that patients with rheumatoid or osteoarthritis can "participate in low-intensity aerobic exercise programs" without aggravating their disease. Low intensity exercise includes things like fast walking and golfing.

"Findings from studies of patients with either rheumatoid arthritis or osteoarthritis who participated in an aerobic exercise program show that the subjects made significant gains, in aerobic capacity, functional status, muscle strength and other aspects of performance," according to the doctors who conducted the study.

The patients also improved in areas "that might have a positive impact on quality of life, including pain tolerance, joint pain, mood, and social activity," say the researchers.

"Despite increasing evidence that regular aerobic exercise yields many benefits for patients with arthritis," the report says, "patients often are advised to curtail physical activity."

But the doctors warn that an inactive approach is not good for most patients because it "may contribute to fatigue, weakness and poor functional performance."

Low aerobic capacity in people with arthritis "is due as much to inactivity" as it is to their disease, the doctors say.

"Aerobic fitness can be improved through participation in a supervised, low-intensity exercise program," according to the report.

Low aerobic capacity is a technical term that means basically the same thing as "being out of shape."

In an evaluation after five years of regular exercise, another researcher found that the arthritis symptoms had not developed as quickly in patients who exercised as in patients who did not.

The people who exercised had also taken less sick time and sick pension from their employers.

Although a stationary exercise bike is convenient and is used in several studies evaluating exercise, bikes are often expensive and people tend to lose interest in them, the doctors caution.

"Swimming, cycling, golf, dancing, gymnastics, fast walking, and jogging ... may be good exercise alternatives," the doctors conclude.

Regular exercise is important, but the sessions don't have to be long.

"As little as 15 minutes of exercise three times per week is sufficient to improve aerobic capacity in arthritis patients with severe limitations," reports T.H. Harkcom in *Arthritis and Rheumatology* (28,1:32).

# Guidelines to aerobic exercise for persons with arthritis

- Only people with mild or moderate arthritis, who can take care of themselves, should be considered for aerobic exercise.

- The best results will occur in people who want to take an active role in their own health care. They need to be motivated to exercise and be willing to work with their doctor's supervision.

- All patients should have an exercise tolerance test, a complete physical, and laboratory studies before they start an exercise program.

- The first six weeks of an exercise program should be supervised by a doctor or physical therapist. Regular check-ups should continue—improvements may change the need for medication.

- Warm-up and cool-down exercises should be taught and faithfully observed.

- Patients should strive to attain 70 percent of their maximal heart rate during their exercise session.

- Proper footwear, with cushioned support to prevent shock, should be worn.

• Ice treatments can be used on aching joints before and after exercise.

• The time of day for exercise should be chosen by the patient and the doctor since some patients have more joint problems in the morning and others experience more discomfort later in the day.

• The doctor should help the person understand the difference between pain normally generated by exercise, and pain related to the arthritis. "Joint pain that lasts longer than one hour after exercise ... should be recognized as a reason to curtail ... activity until the pain subsides."
SOURCE — *Physician and Sportsmedicine*

## Just a little exercise goes a long way

People who completely avoid any physical activity run a 30 percent higher risk of developing coronary heart disease than more active people, according to Martha L. Slattery, a researcher at the University of Utah Medical School.

Slattery found that even the lightest physical activity has a protective, beneficial effect on health in general and the heart in particular. "Small amounts of activity offered protection, and ... little increase in protection is noted for larger amount of physical activity," says the study in the journal *Circulation* (79: 304).

The benefits of exercise were not limited to heart disease

protection — light physical activity reduced death from all causes. "Increasing physical activity, particularly of light-to-moderate intensity, is appropriate to prevent disease and promote health," the authors say.

Since the late 1950s, Slattery and her research team have been studying the health history and leisure-time physical activity of 3,043 white, male railroad workers whose jobs ranged from strenuous physical activity to desk work. Their leisure-time physical activities were classified as light, moderate or intense.

Light activity ranged from walking for pleasure to bowling or raking the lawn. Ballroom dancing and gardening were considered part of the moderate activities, while backpacking, jogging, and snow shoveling, among others, were classified as intense activities.

In a follow-up period that lasted 17 to 20 years, the researchers looked at the leisure-time physical activity habits of the men and compared them to causes of death among those who died. They found that people who reported higher levels of physical activity had lower rates of heart disease. And their findings confirm what other researchers have also seen. "You do not require a lot of activity to get a protective effect," Slattery says.

Statistics show that death rates from diseases of the heart and blood vessels were lower for men who used 1,000 or more calories a week in leisure-time physical activity. That is the equivalent of spending 30 minutes a day in some moderately intense activity, such as playing softball or weeding the garden.

But after taking into account such primary heart disease

risk factors as smoking, high blood pressure and elevated cholesterol, the researchers concluded that "the greatest increase in protection was between those men who were sedentary and those who had some activity," Slattery says.

In other words, desk jockeys and couch potatoes get a great deal of added protection against heart attacks and other diseases just by hoeing weeds in the yard or taking a brisk walk several times a week.

# Heart Problems

## The nation's number one killer

An American dies of cardiovascular disease every 32 seconds. Heart and blood vessel diseases remain the nation's number one killer, claiming an estimated 978,500 Americans in 1986 — one life every 32 seconds, the American Heart Association just announced. By comparison, cancer, the second leading cause of death, claimed almost 466,000 lives. "Cardiovascular diseases killed nearly one million Americans, almost as many as cancer, accidents, pneumonia, influenza and all other causes of death *combined*," reports the AHA's *Heart Facts*.

Heart attacks alone were responsible for 524,100 of the deaths from heart and artery diseases, while strokes accounted for 147,800. High blood pressure, rheumatic heart disease, congenital heart defects, congestive heart failure, and other cardiovascular disease accounted for the other deaths.

Despite this appalling death toll, there are encouraging signs, the AHA says. From 1976 to 1986, the death rate from coronary heart disease fell 27.9 percent, while death from stroke dropped 40.2 percent. Death rates from rheumatic fever, congenital heart disease and high blood pressure also continued to decline. 1986 is the most recent year for which death rates and statistics are available.

Of the total U. S. population of about 241 million in 1986, about 66 million Americans had at least one form of cardiovascular disease. Some 60,130,000 had high blood pressure, by far the most common cardiovascular disease and a risk factor for both stroke and heart attack, AHA warns.

About 1.5 million Americans will suffer a heart attack in 1989, and more than 500,000 of them will die, the AHA predicts. About 60 percent of those deaths (or more than 300,000) will occur before the victims reach a hospital. Fifty percent of heart attack victims wait more than two hours before getting to an emergency room.

Most of the more than 6,000 general hospitals in the United States have coronary care capability, which can reduce in-hospital deaths by about 30 percent. The AHA estimates that the cost of heart and artery diseases in 1989 will be $88.2 billion, a figure that includes the cost of hospital and nursing home care ($56.3 billion), lost productivity ($15 billion), physicians and nursing services ($12.5 billion) and medication ($4.4 billion).

Other statistics from *Heart Facts* :

- Each day the average heart beats 100,000 times and pumps close to 2,000 gallons of blood.

• Atherosclerosis or "hardening of the arteries" was a major contributor to the estimated 61,900 heart attack and stroke deaths in 1986.

• About 2,470,000 Americans suffer from angina, chest pain associated with coronary artery disease. About 300,000 new cases occur each year.

• Approximately 45 percent of all heart attack victims are under age 65, and 5 percent are under age 40.

• Three to four million Americans are thought to have episodes of "silent ischemia," which damage the heart without causing noticeable pain.

• In U.S. adults aged 18-74, high blood pressure affects 38 percent of black males, 33 percent of white males, 39 percent of black females and 25 percent of white females.

• Coronary artery bypass grafts increased to 284,000 in 1986, up from 230,000 in 1985. Balloon angioplasties— where a balloon-tipped catheter is guided to a narrowed artery segment, inflated and the artery widened — increased from 82,000 in 1985 to 133,000 in 1986.

• There were 1,418 human heart transplants performed in the U.S. in 1987, almost nine times as many as in 1983.

A report in the *American Journal of Clinical Nutrition* (49,5:993) outlines how your diet can mean the difference between healthy maturity and lingering illnesses. Many studies concerning diet and your heart generally show that excess fat and sugar are risk factors for heart attack and artery disease.

One study examined diet and heart-disease deaths for 30 countries and found that fat, sugar, animal protein and total calories increased heart disease among men aged 55 to 59. Most experts recommend a balanced diet that cuts back on the amount of calories gotten from fat and cholesterol-containing foods. Cold-water fish provide a good source of omega-3 fatty acids, one kind of fat that seems to be good for your heart and circulatory system.

Starches and vegetable proteins are beneficial, according to the journal report. Also, exercise more, and try to drop some weight, especially any "spare tire" of excess pounds around the middle.

Other risk factors include stress, smoking, high cholesterol and blood pressure and a sedentary (non-exercising) lifestyle.

## New health risks for smokers

A new study of twins finds that smoking is a "strong factor" in the development of carotid atherosclerosis, the hardening and narrowing of the large arteries that supply blood to the head. The study of 49 pairs of identical twins in Finland shows that the association of smoking with carotid atherosclerosis was "highly significant," even after statistically adjusting for age, cholesterol level, blood pressure and other potentially confounding factors, according to the report in *Circulation* (80:10-16).

In each of the 49 pairs studied, one twin was a non-smoker or at least never had smoked daily, and the other was a smoker or ex-smoker. The average life-long dose of the smoking twins was 20 "package-years"— they had smoked the equivalent of one package every day for 20 years. That contrasts sharply with the twins who were classified as non-smokers, who had smoked less than five packages (100 cigarettes) in their entire lives.

Because of difficulties in performing well-controlled experiments on human populations, researchers often turn to identical twins who are, in a sense, "natural experiments." Both twins have the same genetic makeup, thus limiting a major variable and giving researchers a better opportunity to study the effects of lifestyle and environmental factors such as smoking.

Using ultrasound in external examinations, the scientists measured "plaques" in the carotid arteries of the twins. Plaque is a fatty deposit attached to a wall of a blood vessel. Studies by others have shown that smoking is associated with development of plaques in the abdominal aorta, in the heart arteries and in major arteries in the legs, say the Finnish researchers.

In the 49 pairs included in the analyses, narrowing of the carotids was found in nine pairs — nine of the smoking twins and two of their non-smoking co-twins, the researchers report. The total area of artery-narrowing plaques in the carotids was more than three times larger in the smoking twins.

The inner layer of the carotid arteries was thicker in the smoking twins, the study says. Both total area and thickness correlated with the dose of smoking — the more one smoked, the worse the plugging effect. Based on this 12-year study, the researchers concluded, "The smoking twins are at a significantly higher risk of coronary heart disease than their non-smoking co-twins."

For us non-twins, the study demonstrates that smoking greatly raises the risk of plaque plugs in vital neck arteries. Increased plaque, in turn, raises the risk of stroke and hemorrhage due to weakened or blocked arteries.

## An early warning sign of heart and artery disease

If you are a middle-aged man who is frequently out of breath, you may be a prime candidate for a heart attack, suggests a report in *Modern Medicine* (57,9:139).

In a British study, nearly four out of every ten men who had breathlessness but no signs of heart disease at their initial screening exam had developed angina, suffered a heart attack or died within five years. By contrast, only one out of every twelve men (fewer than one in ten) without breathlessness at screening developed angina or other heart problems during the same period.

Angina is severe pain in the chest and arms brought on by blocked heart arteries. It indicates serious, even potentially fatal, heart disease.

"A strong association was also found between breathlessness and silent electrocardiographic evidence of [coronary artery disease], even in men with no other evidence of [the disease] at screening," say the authors of a report from the British Regional Heart Study, a study involving 7,735 British men 40 to 59 years old. The likelihood of eventual heart disease seemed to be linked directly to the severity of the breathlessness, the report says. In other words, the more out of breath you are, the more likely you are to come down with heart problems.

Check with your doctor if even minor exertion causes you to puff and pant for breath. The doctor may recommend immediate steps you can take to begin lowering your heart attack risk, including changing to a healthier diet and getting into better physical shape.

## The newest heart-disease risk factor

High levels of insulin in the blood may be a silent heart-disease risk factor for 25 percent of the trim and otherwise healthy people in the U.S., according to a report in *Science News* (136,12:184).

This was confirmed by a report recently presented to the American Diabetes Association by Dr. Annick Fontbonne, a researcher at the French National Institute of Health and Medical Research, who stated, "Our studies indicate that the earliest marker of a higher risk of coronary heart disease mortality is an elevation of stimulated plasma insulin level."

Scientists believe that a long-term excess of insulin "silently damages the cardiovascular system," although how remains a mystery. "Some speculate that high insulin levels may directly damage the artery wall, leading to a buildup of fat that narrows the vessel."

Insulin resistance occurs when the pancreas produces enough insulin — a hormone that directs cells to take up glucose (sugar) from the blood — but the body does not respond well. Blood sugar levels rise, and the pancreas then churns out more insulin to meet the body's demand.

Type II diabetes (also called non-insulin-dependent diabetes) results from high blood sugar levels. It affects 10 million Americans — generally, overweight people over age 40, who are "two to four times as likely as nondiabetics to develop heart disease," according to the report.

Not all insulin-resistant people are diabetic. Dr. Gerald M. Reaven, of Stanford University School of Medicine, has researched insulin resistance for more than 20 years and has identified what he calls "syndrome X," a series of heart-disease risk factors affecting insulin-resistant — but otherwise healthy — people.

The risk factors are the following:

- High blood pressure
- High triglycerides (a form of fat in the bloodstream)
- Decreased high-density-lipoprotein (HDL) cholesterol— "good"
- High cholesterol

Although Type I (insulin-dependent) diabetics have a

definite heart-disease risk, Dr. Reaven is having a difficult time convincing diabetes specialists that people who are insulin-resistant — whether diabetic or not — are at risk as well.

The syndrome X theory is controversial, yet may explain why people in countries such as India and Pakistan have lower cholesterol levels but greater incidence of heart disease than people in other countries.

Many researchers believe syndrome X is hereditary, but further research will try to determine whether environmental factors, such as obesity, trigger it.

Studies in France and Italy have confirmed the syndrome X theory, which has also been put to the test at the Pittsburgh School of Medicine.

There researchers studied "489 healthy, white, premenopausal women aged 42 to 52" and found "an increasing risk of heart disease as blood levels of insulin rise."

The women had an average total cholesterol level of 185, considered normal. "Women with the highest blood insulin levels proved the most likely to have high blood pressure, elevated triglycerides and decreased HDL cholesterol values," according to the report.

Insulin levels increased as body mass (weight in kilograms divided by height in meters) increased, but the "study doesn't offer any hints as to which came first, the increased body weight or higher insulin levels, reports *Medical World News* (30,16:14)."

Body mass is a significant heart-disease risk factor, but fat distribution — namely, upper-body obesity — is also a signal, Swedish researchers report in *Medical World News*. "Abdominal fat cells are metabolically more active ... and release more fatty acid." Although upper-body obesity occurs primarily in men, women with similar amounts of abdominal fat would have the same risk, researchers said.

Other studies have identified insulin levels as a risk factor for men. In a report recently presented to the American Diabetes Association, Israeli researcher Michaela Modan stated, "Tests for insulin resistance could be an even earlier indicator of coronary heart disease risk than cholesterol and other blood lipid evaluations." In Modan's study, 1,258 males were evaluated for body weight, blood pressure levels, heart disease, glucose and insulin response. "As expected, the rate of hyperinsulinemia (high levels of insulin in the blood) was 3.3-fold more frequent in individuals who had either glucose intolerance, obesity, or hypertension ... than among those who did not," says Dr. Modan.

However, in men with hyperinsulinemia, rates of heart disease in men with glucose intolerance, obesity or high blood pressure were over four times that of normal controls — 10.2 percent versus 2.4 percent. Dr. Modan suggests that finding a simple test for insulin resistance might pave the way for mass screening of people for this "red flag" indicator of heart disease.

The technique used in the study was an oral glucose tolerance test. The test involved taking repeated blood samples over a two-hour period. This "crude method" is effective for the study, but is not simple enough for mass screenings, she says. "Furthermore, although hypertension (high blood pressure) may be an independent risk factor, it presents a three-fold greater risk when it occurs in the presence of hyperinsulinemia," she says. In fat people, weight loss and physical activity usually can help reduce or eliminate hyperinsuline-mia.

## Aspirin every other day reduces risk of first heart attack

In the United States alone, heart attacks strike over 1.5 million people each year, killing about half of them. Taking a 325-milligram aspirin tablet every other day can sharply reduce the risk of first heart attacks in healthy men, especially those over age 50, according to a major medical study published in *The New England Journal of Medicine* (321,3:129).

The aspirin therapy resulted in a 47 percent reduction in risk of a first heart attack among 22,000 male doctors, says the final report of the Physician's Health Study, which was sponsored by the National Institutes of Health.

The Food and Drug Administration (FDA) must review the results of this study, since aspirin hasn't received government approval as a medicine to prevent first heart attacks.

Daily aspirin in doses from 160 to 325 milligrams, when prescribed by a physician, currently is FDA-approved to help prevent second heart attacks and recurring unstable angina.

Buffered aspirin was used in the study, but regular aspirin or enteric (coated) aspirin would also be effective, the researchers say. However, acetaminophen (like Tylenol) does not have the same effect.

The researchers tested several different doses of aspirin

and found that one aspirin every second day was the most effective. An aspirin every day (for people without previous heart problems) did not increase its protective effect, but did increase unwanted side effects like stomach bleeding and indigestion.

It is important to remember that in healthy people and heart patients, aspirin therapy does not treat the plaque buildup and artery disease that causes heart attacks. Aspirin only reduces the blood's ability to clot.

Aspirin should not be used as a substitute for other prevention therapies for heart attacks, cautions FDA commissioner Dr. Frank E. Young.

All known ways of fighting artery disease — like not smoking, reducing fat intake, lowering high blood pressure and exercising — should be carefully followed, the report says.

Dr. Lawrence Cohen from Yale University School of Medicine, a member of the research committee overseeing the study, is optimistic about the report. But Dr. Cohen cautions that using aspirin to prevent heart attacks must be a decision made between doctor and patient.

Aspirin acts like a blood thinner, reducing its ability to clot. That could pose serious problems for people who already are taking blood-thinning medicine, have bleeding ulcers, or have recently undergone surgery. In an *NEJM* editorial (321,3,:183), the journal says, "Aspirin should be used cautiously, if at all, in patients with diabetic retinopathy or poorly controlled hypertension."

Incidentally, that same clinical study also sought to discover whether 50 milligrams of beta carotene given every other day to this same group of 22,000 male doctors had any effect on preventing cancer. No findings have been announced about the parallel beta carotene study. The aspirin part of the study was ended three years earlier than scheduled because of the dramatic results ascribed to aspirin for preventing heart attacks.

## Ear crease may be an early warning signal of a heart attack

A diagonal crease across your earlobe at a 45-degree downward angle toward your shoulder may be an early warning sign of a potentially fatal heart attack, according to reports in *Modern Medicine* (57,10:126) and *British Heart Journal* (611,4:361).

You might think we're pulling your, uh..., ears.

But, scientists have been studying the amazing ear-crease phenomenon since 1973 — with inconclusive results until this research report.

In the latest study, they found telltale ear creases in both fat and skinny people who died from sudden heart attacks, so weight wasn't a factor.

The common denominator was sudden death, often in people who apparently didn't know how sick they were.

In the current study, researchers randomly selected 303 people whose cause of death was unknown before autopsy.

They found diagonal ear creases in 72 percent of the dead men and 67 percent of the deceased women.

Men with diagonal ear creases were 55 percent more likely to die of heart disease than men without ear creases.

The risk was even greater for non-diabetic women (1.74 times more likely to die of heart disease).

Interestingly, ear creases did not predict death from heart disease in diabetic women.

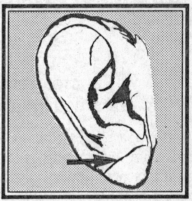

· Those with ear creases generally don't get them until after age 50, the reports say.

Fatness apparently does not influence whether people have ear creases, researchers say, because both fat and thin people have them in roughly equal numbers.

However, people with heart disease seem to develop the creases, regardless of their age, they add.

The alarming thing was the link between ear creases and unexpected death.

Many people in this study had died suddenly from heart attacks, but had no history of heart disease, the researchers say.

In this group, earlobe creases alone were a greater predictor of sudden death from heart attack than known risk factors, such as previous heart disease, the studies report.

That fact has led researchers to speculate that some doctors may be missing severe heart disease cases among some middle-aged and elderly people.

If that's the case, help yourself by checking your ears for diagonal creases.

If there's a crease, tell your doctor about the crease and about these studies.

## Fish oil and heart surgery

Recent studies suggest that fish oil taken before and after two very different kinds of surgery can have highly beneficial effects. In one study, fish oil seemed to help keep arteries unclogged after "balloon" surgery. In another, fish oil apparently helped prevent the spread of cancer cells that escaped after operations.

An extremely high intake of fish oil can "dramatically improve" the results of coronary angioplasty, popularly known as "balloon" surgery, according to one new study at the Washington Hospital Center. Usually about one-third of arteries opened with angioplasty get clogged up again with cholesterol and plaque within six months. But Dr. Mark R. Milner said his research suggests that taking large doses of fish oil for just six months can cut that failure rate in half.

Fish oil seemed to help patients after another kind of surgery, as well. A Harvard Medical School study suggested that highly purified fish oil supplements helped prevent spread of cancer cells that may escape during and after surgical operations to remove cancerous tissue.

Dr. George Blackburn of Harvard, who's also chief of

nutrition support at New England Deaconess Hospital, said the fish oil supplements were given to cancer patients a week before surgery. Following surgery, the patients continued taking the fish oil for three to six months. Blackburn noted lower rates of cancer spread, known as metastasis, in those who took fish oil.

Both doctors have a very conservative approach to fish oil therapy for all but these two classes of surgery patients. Milner advised against taking fish oil capsules for any other reason, because, he said, the long-term effects are still unknown. "I never give fish oil supplements to any of my patients unless they are having coronary angioplasty," he said. Blackburn recommended eating deep-water fish four or five times a week, rather than taking fish oil capsules.

In the fish oil study on heart patients, 194 persons were randomly assigned to two groups following successful angioplasty. One group took nine fish oil capsules per day for six months after the procedure. Each capsule contained a total of 4.5 grams of omega-3 fatty acids. That's about the daily equivalent of the fish oil in two cans of sardines.

The other group got no fish oil, but patients in both groups were told to eat low-fat, low-cholesterol diets. Both groups received the same post-operative therapy. Nurses trained in diet therapy called each patient monthly to provide counseling and to evaluate if the patients were sticking to their strict diet.

"Dietary compliance was equally good in both groups of patients," Milner noted. "They really tried to stick with a strict low-cholesterol diet." Patients' cholesterol intake was restricted to 100 milligrams per day, and dietary fat was limited to 25 percent of their total calories.

By the end of six months, 35.4 percent of people who didn't take the fish oil showed signs that their dilated heart arteries had narrowed again. However, the recurrence rate in the fish oil group was only about 19 percent, Milner reported.

During the study, eleven patients stopped taking the high doses of fish oil because of disagreeable, but not dangerous, side effects including flatulence and other mild digestive problems. Milner said that most patients were willing to tolerate the side effects in order to possibly lower their risk of having a repeat angioplasty or needing bypass surgery.

Coronary angioplasty is less invasive than heart bypass surgery because it does not involve cutting open the chest cavity. Instead, the surgeon cuts into a leg or arm artery and inserts a catheter with a tiny balloon on the tip. He threads the narrow catheter through the circulatory system until its tip reaches the portion of the heart artery that is narrowed by fatty "plaque." Then the doctor inflates the balloon, squashing the plaque against the artery wall and enlarging the inner diameter of the blood vessel. Several blockages can be opened during the procedure.

An estimated 184,000 Americans had angioplasty in 1987. Since the use of angioplasty began about a decade ago, scientists have been searching for a drug to reduce the procedure's failure rate.

Aspirin has proven to be helpful in reducing the numbers of heart attacks that happened during or soon after angioplasty. But aspirin doesn't seem to make a significant difference in reducing the six-month reclogging rate, known as "restenosis," said Milner, who is assistant professor of medicine at George Washington University.

Milner's findings are similar to the results of a smaller study of 82 patients at the Dallas VA Medical Center, reported in the *New England Journal of Medicine*. Milner said several research teams are doing comparable studies to confirm these results.

Fish oil seems to suppress the inflammatory response that follows an injury, Milner said. In angioplasty, the inner wall of the artery is sometimes injured by the balloon catheter.

If the injured area heals rapidly, excess inflammation, scar tissue and blood clots may combine to clog the artery again. Fish oil seems to slow the unwanted speedy healing process and to prevent the inflammation and scarring. It also seems to reduce the tendency of blood platelets to form clots at the once-clogged site.

## Coffee and caffeine: how much is too much?

If you're worried about your cholesterol levels or suffer from cardiovascular disease, put down your cup of coffee and take note. Research indicates that drinking one to five cups of caffeinated coffee every day nearly doubles your risk of heart disease and strokes, compared with non-coffee drinkers, according to *U.S. Pharmacist* (14,6:28). Six cups a day of the regular brew increases your risk 2.5 times, the report says.

A "safe" daily intake of caffeine is about 200 milligrams (less than one-hundredth of one ounce), according to the report. But one regular cup of coffee contains at least 170 milligrams.

Excess caffeine can provoke arrhythmia, an irregular heartbeat. That can be dangerous for some people. Too much caffeine also seems to be linked to increased levels of blood cholesterol, which in turn can be very bad for your heart and arteries.

In one eight-week study, patients with existing heart rhythm problems got worse after taking the equivalent of three to five cups of caffeinated coffee each day, says a report in *American Family Physician* (39,6:214).

Researchers haven't managed to tag coffee with directly causing cancer. But, they point out, heavy users of caffeine also tend to be heavy smokers.

Tobacco smoking has been established to be a proven, direct cause of lung cancer. As for other cancers, "It appears that coffee drinkers are marginally more likely to develop bladder cancer than abstainers," says the *U.S. Pharmacist* report.

A 1981 study suggested a link between caffeine and cancer of the pancreas, but that has not been confirmed in other studies.

Coffee is the major source of caffeine for most Americans. Just two cups a day can put you over "the safe limit," defined in this report as 200 milligrams.

But did you know that a cup of drip or percolated coffee has nearly 80 milligrams of caffeine more than the same cup filled with instant coffee?

If you don't like decaffeinated coffee (which contains five milligrams of caffeine), try instant coffee instead to cut your daily intake, the report suggests.

Some other caffeine counts to note are the following:

Brewed tea, 6 oz. cup — 50 milligrams of caffeine
Instant tea, 6 oz. cup — 30 milligrams
Cola drinks, 12 oz. — 30 to 50 milligrams
Hot cocoa, 6 oz. cup — 2 to 8 milligrams
Sweet dark chocolate, 1 oz. — 5 to 35 milligrams
Chocolate desserts — 10 milligrams

Note: pain relief medication also can contain caffeine. One Excedrin tablet, for example, contains 65 milligrams of caffeine.

People who consume excess caffeine — 500 to 600 milligrams a day — may experience caffeinism, or "coffee nerves," and become addicted. You may be suffering from caffeinism if you have several symptoms like these: restlessness, insomnia, flushed face, stomach upset, nervousness and irregular heartbeat.

Cutting back from large daily doses of caffeine all at once may cause you to experience severe withdrawal symptoms, like throbbing headache, fatigue, irritability and anxiety.

Try to avoid "self-medicating" yourself with a cup of coffee. That's a step in the wrong direction, doctors say. Instead, try to cut down your caffeine habit gradually, rather than quitting "cold turkey."

## Which is worse — a fat stomach or fat hips?

A fat stomach, commonly known as a "spare tire" or a

"beer belly," is more dangerous to your health than fat hips or legs. Abdominal (or stomach) obesity is linked with an increased risk of stroke in men and heart failure in both sexes, according to researchers from Boston University who studied a group of 4,500 adults for 20 years as part of the Framingham Study.

"As the ratio of abdominal girth to height increases, so does the risk of developing cardiovascular disease," said Dr. Joseph Stokes III, professor of medicine at Boston University.

"Just looking at overall weight didn't predict which people would develop cardiovascular disease or die," Stokes explained. "Abdominal obesity was a stronger predictor."

Heart failure was the complication most strongly associated with abdominal obesity, according to Stokes. For each 2.5 inches of fat, another 10 to 12 people per 1,000 developed heart failure.

The thickness of the skin-fold under the shoulder blade, an estimator of upper body fat, appears to be another independent indicator of risk, noted William B. Kannel, another researcher involved in the Framingham Heart Study.

At this point, researchers can only theorize why they believe excess stomach fat is more damaging than other fat. Some think that since the blood flows through this fatty tissue directly to the liver, the organ that secretes and removes cholesterol from the blood, the fat causes more heart problems. Others suggest that the fat cells in the stomach may be regulated in a different way than those in the buttocks and thighs.

Stroke often causes paralysis or other severe neurological problems after the blood supply is cut off to an area of the brain. Congestive heart failure results when a weakened heart muscle can't deliver enough oxygen to the body.

## Poor dental health may be a risk factor for heart disease

According to new research from Finland, poor dental health may be a risk factor for developing heart disease, the *British Medical Journal* (298,6676:779) reports. In two separate studies, people with heart disease "had worse dental health than controls" even when other risk factors for heart disease were excluded, Dr. Kimmo Mattila explains in the journal.

"Little is known about the long-term effects of chronic low grade bacterial infections" that are associated with cavities and gum disease, says the journal. The authors suggest that poisons produced by these bacteria in the mouth may have a harmful effect on the heart.

## Before you have surgery, check the hospital's track record

If you are scheduled to have an operation, you will want to know something the hospital won't automatically reveal to you — the death rates for that kind of surgical procedure at that hospital.

In major surgery, as in most important things in life, practice makes, if not perfect, then at least less dangerous.

Ask a hospital official these questions, and don't be satisfied until you have a full and complete answer to each question:

(1) How many times during the past 12 months has my particular kind of operation been performed at this hospital?

(2) How many people have died during or following such a procedure at this hospital?

(3) What are the comparable rates for this surgery for specific hospitals in this area?

If you can't get this information from your chosen hospital, you should check with the government agency responsible for licensing hospitals in your state for answers to these questions.

Other sources are the state and federal agencies responsible for making or auditing Medicare and Medicaid payments.

The point is this: if you must have a heart operation, a hospital that performs 200 open-heart surgeries a year is probably a better choice than one that performs only 25 such operations in the same period. The same goes for the surgical team.

Death rates for identical surgical procedures also can give clues to which hospitals you may want to avoid.

But remember — you have to aggressively seek such information well before you are wheeled into the operating room. Most likely, it won't be volunteered to you.

# Hemorrhoids

## Reading and hemorrhoids

If you read during a leisurely bathroom break, you are likely to develop painful hemorrhoids. That's the apparent connection revealed in a study reported in *The Lancet* (1, 8628:54).

"We found that patients with hemorrhoids tend to spend longer defecating and also are more likely to read and strain while defecating than are patients without hemorrhoids," the researchers said.

While this subject may strike some as indelicate, an attack of hemorrhoids is one of the most common conditions suffered by Americans. Many millions of dollars are spent every year on over-the-counter remedies, visits to doctors and more drastic surgical solutions.

The study suggests that many sufferers may bring the problem on themselves, mostly through poor bowel habits.

# Osteoporosis

## How caffeine affects your bones

Everyone loses some bone mass as part of the aging process, especially after the age of 40. But for some, it becomes a much more serious problem than for others. Here's some news about what you can do to protect your bones and to avoid the dangers of osteoporosis.

First, the abnormal amount of bone loss, known as osteoporosis, is the result of calcium in the bones being drawn out into the blood and excreted in the urine. The bones become brittle, the amount of bone mass is reduced, and the strength of remaining bone is weakened. The condition can cause loss of height or a humped back, especially in women past the menopause, and usually is first diagnosed because of a fracture of the hip, wrist, or spinal vertebrae.

So, we need to keep this valuable calcium from being leached out of our bones. Several studies have shown the negative effect of coffee in causing bone loss. But new research has just confirmed that it is the caffeine in coffee that causes calcium loss. Put simply, the more caffeine you drink, the more calcium is driven out of your bones.

At Mt. Saint Vincent University in Halifax, Nova Scotia, researcher Susan Whiting tested different properties of coffee in animals to determine exactly what causes the loss of calcium. Whiting demonstrated that it is the caffeine in coffee, not the diuretic effect, that takes calcium from the body.

In another study, Dr. Linda K. Massey reported that caffeinated-coffee drinkers lose twice as much calcium as people who drink decaffeinated coffee. In her work at Washington State University, Massey found that caffeine causes calcium to be excreted in urine.

Since many coffee drinkers are not getting enough calcium to begin with, drinking coffee containing caffeine is making their problem worse, Massey believes. If you must drink coffee, use decaffeinated coffee with lots of milk. The additional milk will help replace some of the calcium that the body needs, reports *Prevention* (39:5).

## High risk factors for osteoporosis

- Being female
- Being Caucasian
- Family history of osteoporosis or hip fractures
- Slender build
- Being inactive

- Low muscle mass
- Early menopause
- Being past menopause
- Fair or translucent skin
- Cigarette smoking
- Low calcium intake
- High alcohol consumption
- Drinking lots of soft drinks
- Consuming large amounts of caffeine
- High protein diet
- Taking thyroid hormones
- Long-term treatment with steroids for arthritis, asthma or other diseases
- Having anorexia nervosa, a serious loss of appetite

Sources: *Modern Medicine* (57,3:114) and *The Encyclopedia of Top Secret Ways to Defeat Old Age* (FC&A Publishing)

## Study says calcium needed throughout life

To get the best protection against osteoporosis, you should make sure you get recommended amounts of calcium in your diet beginning early in life, a new study revealed in the *Journal of the American Medical Association* (260:3150).

Women who maintained high-calcium diets throughout their lives, as children, adolescents, and reproductive women, have the highest bone density, according to the study. "Swallowing calcium pills at 50 years of age probably is not going to make your bones thicker," one researcher said.

"In our analysis, the only group in which a protective effect of calcium could be observed was in women who reported both a high milk consumption during periods of growth and development, as well as currently," the report concluded.

Damage from osteoporosis is usually permanent. The most common treatments include heat, drugs for the pain, a back brace and rest. Rest, combined with moderate exercise like walking, helps keep the muscles in shape to support the weak bone structure. Since damage from osteoporosis is difficult to repair, prevention should be a life-long goal.

## Study shows it's never too late to reduce the risk of osteoporosis

Regular exercise like walking, jogging or climbing stairs, combined with adequate calcium intake, can help reduce the risk of osteoporosis in women past the age of menopause, reports the *Annals of Internal Medicine* (108,6:824).

Researchers studied a group of women between 55 and 70 years of age. The women exercised three times a week for 50-60 minutes each session. Each woman also took 1,500 milli-grams of calcium daily. "The response to exercise was posi-tive for at least 22 months" (the length of the study), explained Gail Dalsky, the researcher who led the study at Washington University School of Medicine in St. Louis. The density of the bones actually increased, she said. However, when regular exercise stopped or was reduced, the bone density returned to its pre-exercise condition, even with calcium supplementation. The study suggests that regular exercise may fight bone loss in women over 50.

Osteoporosis afflicts approximately five million Americans — most are elderly women past menopause. The disease is an abnormal loss of bone that leads to brittle bones, hip and wrist fractures and curving of the spine. Helping to strengthen the bones by increasing the bone mass helps to reduce the risk of fractures.

Dalsky stressed that weight-bearing exercise should supplement, not replace, other known treatments for osteoporosis like estrogen-replacement therapy and additional calcium. "Exercise can usually be safely added to such therapies, but it can't be substituted for them," Dalsky says in another report of her study in *The Physician and Sportsmedicine* (17,2:48).

Other studies have shown that weight-bearing exercise helps the bones to grow stronger and more dense. Weight-bearing exercise is physical activity in which the bones have to support body weight, including aerobics, dancing, walking, jogging, hiking, rope jumping, or tennis. Weight-bearing exercise may be combined with other types of exercise like swimming, bicycling, and rowing to provide a variety of activities that will keep the exercise sessions interesting.

Until now, doctors did not know if exercise after menopause would just stop the bones from deteriorating farther, or if it would actually help to increase the density of the bones.

# Smoking linked to bone loss

Researchers at Argonne National Laboratory in Illinois report yet another link between osteoporosis and smoking. Osteoporosis is a long-term loss of bone material, causing stooped shoulders and bent spines, especially in older women. They discovered that high levels of the poisonous element cadmium promoted bone loss in both animal and laboratory tests. Cadmium is found in tobacco in cigarettes. "Bone loss was greatest at cadmium levels roughly equivalent to those found in smokers' blood," according to a report in *Medical World News* (30,3:18).

# Take steps to prevent osteoporosis

The best way to manage osteoporosis is to prevent it from developing. Since osteoporosis develops silently over many years, proper diet and exercise throughout your life are extremely important.

- Adequate calcium. The daily diet should include foods that are high in calcium like dairy products (including milk, cheese, and yogurt), dark green leafy vegetables (like collards, turnip greens, spinach and broccoli), salmon, sardines, oysters, and tofu.

- Adequate vitamin D. Vitamin-fortified milk, cereals,

saltwater fish, liver and daily sunshine are good sources of this vitamin.

• Adequate manganese. Manganese is an important mineral found in whole-grain products, fruits (especially bananas), vegetables (especially legumes), eggs, liver and other organ meats.

• Adequate exercise. Walking, jogging, dancing, bicycling, aerobics, rowing, hiking, rope jumping, tennis and other exercise in which the bones have to support body weight, helps promote bone growth.

• With your doctor, consider estrogen replacement therapy during menopause. When estrogen replacement therapy is started right after women stop menstruating, hip and wrist fractures can be reduced as much as 60 percent.

• Avoid smoking, alcoholic beverages, drinks containing caffeine, soft drinks, meat, and high protein foods.

Source: National Institutes of Health and *Stand Tall* by Notelovitz and Ware

# Nutrition

## Health problems caused
## by poor nutrition

For people over age 50, more health problems are caused by poor nutrition and lack of exercise than by aging alone, indicates a report in *Geriatrics* (44,6:57). Many older people fail to get even the official recommended daily allowances of vitamins and minerals necessary for good health.

For example, of those over age 60, more than half the men and more than seven out of every 10 women don't get enough folic acid (a B vitamin) and vitamin B6, according to the *Geriatrics* report.

In that same age group, about five of every 10 men and six of every 10 women fall short of getting enough vitamin D.

Smaller percentages in that age group have problems getting enough zinc, calcium, vitamin B12 and vitamin A.

There are many reasons. First, many people don't know

what the recommended daily allowances are. Secondly, they don't know what foods to eat or drink to meet the requirements. And in a few cases, aging digestive systems don't process certain vitamins and minerals as well as in younger years.

Although researchers are still studying the particular nutritional needs of older Americans, moderation seems to be the key to good health. Maintain a low-salt, low-fat, well-balanced diet by eating a variety of fruits, vegetables, whole grains and lean meats. Limit your intake of alcohol, and talk to your physician about an exercise program. Regular exercise will help you keep up a healthy appetite.

The foods you eat — and how much you eat — have a big impact on your risk of developing certain diseases, especially heart disease, according to a report in the *American Journal of Clinical Nutrition* (49,5:995).

"Diet, through calorie, salt, alcohol, and fat intake, plays a fundamental role in the development of cardiovascular disease," the report says. Excess amounts of meat, eggs, animal protein and animal fat are related to heart disease, and excess salt and alcohol are related to hypertension. Obesity has been linked with stroke, liver and heart diseases, and problems during surgery.

Vitamins alone won't keep you healthy, and excess doses can be toxic. Therefore, discuss with your doctor your plans for taking vitamin and mineral supplements.

"By taking a vitamin pill, people think they are maintaining their health and are distracted from controlling the factors that will have the most impact on their health — total fat, calories and cholesterol," says a report in *Archives of Internal Medicine* (149,6:1254).

## Build a 'foundation' diet for good health

You may think it's "too late" to change your eating habits, but that is not so. Changing your eating habits today will go a long way toward promoting good health tomorrow, regardless of your age.

Take these tips from nutritionist Nancy Clark, who outlines a "foundation diet" in *Senior Patient* (1,5:95). She encourages you to eat more of these good foods:

**Dairy products** — Even if you're watching cholesterol, don't eliminate dairy foods entirely, she advises. Choose nonfat (rather than low-fat) products, which have all the vitamins and minerals you need without the fat. You should have three servings of dairy products each day.

Try a cup of nonfat yogurt with fruit with lunch or add powdered milk to mashed potatoes. A hefty scoop of cottage cheese has only 130 milligrams of calcium but a whopping 20 grams of protein (equivalent to a quarter-pound hamburger before it's cooked).

**Fruits** — Orange and grapefruit juices are more nutritious than other fruit juices, such as apple, grape and cranberry — and they  lower in calories, too. A six-ounce glass of orange juice will provide your daily requirement of vitamin C. But eating the whole fruit is better than drinking a glass of juice, according to the nutritionist.

Bananas are potassium-rich and have only about 100 calories — a good afternoon snack. Spread peanut butter on top for extra protein.

**Vegetables** — Choose dark, colorful vegetables — romaine lettuce, spinach, green peppers, broccoli and carrots. One carrot — whether cooked or grated into a salad — will also provide the recommended daily allowance of vitamin A or its equivalent in beta carotene, the report says. Celery, cucumbers, onions and radishes have a greater "crunch factor" but are not as nutritious.

Another way to get your RDA of vitamin C is to eat "one stalk of cooked broccoli, half a green pepper, two medium tomatoes or a spinach salad." Avoid canned or processed tomatoes, which are high in sodium. Tomato juice and sauce are fine and "are as nutritious as fresh tomatoes." Winter squash is high in vitamin A and potassium.

Potatoes are nutrient-rich (potassium, fiber and vitamin C), can be prepared many ways and are better for you than rice or noodles. Potatoes are *not* fattening; what you put on them is. Avoid butter, sour cream and gravies. Try instead a baked potato with a butter substitute or a little skim milk and "mash" the potato.

Don't overcook vegetables. They will retain more nutrients if they're microwaved or steamed rather than boiled.

**Starches** — Generally, darker breads are more nutritious than refined white breads. Whole-wheat, bran and rye breads are fiber-rich. Try a slice with a thin spread of peanut butter.

Freeze bread to keep it fresh; it takes only a few minutes for slices to thaw.

Bran cereals are good sources of fiber and iron and help lower cholesterol. "Look for the words 'enriched' or fortified on the labels," the nutritionist suggests. To get a healthy start in the morning, try bran cereal with skim milk, a banana and a glass of orange juice.

**Meat and fish** — Nutritionists recommend two weekly servings of fish, which keeps your heart healthy and is easy to prepare. "Put the fish in a shallow pan, add a little water, cover and cook over medium heat for about five minutes until it flakes easily when pierced with a fork," Nancy Clark says.

Choose extra-lean ground beef and turkey — good sources of protein, vitamins, iron and zinc. Limit beef to three four-ounce servings a week. Commercially prepared turkey usually has more fat and calories than turkey prepared at home.

**Treats** — "Fig newtons, raisin squares, animal crackers and gingersnaps are acceptable treats because they're lower in saturated fats than most desserts and offer slightly more nutritional value than chocolate chip cookies," she says in the report.

## Yogurt may improve your health

Remember when only dieters ate yogurt? The many brands of yogurt on the supermarket shelves and the frozen yogurt

stores popping up across the country are signs that times —
and tastes — have changed. Yogurt is *in*.

This sudden popularity of yogurt is more than a fad. It's
based on years of medical research that suggests that for many
people, fermented milk products like yogurt can help keep
them in good health.

Yogurt is a good source of calcium, especially for people
who have trouble digesting lactose (a milk sugar) and thus
cannot drink milk. Yogurt contains less lactose than milk,
which makes it easier to digest. Easily digestible calcium is
important in preventing osteoporosis, a bone loss disease that
afflicts some middle-aged and elderly women.

Fermented milk products are beneficial in treating other
conditions, too, says a report in *The American Journal of
Clinical Nutrition* (49,4:675). Indigestion, high levels of
cholesterol in the blood, bowel irregularity, high blood pressure and even food poisoning have been known to yield to a
diet that includes fermented milk.

Although researchers don't know the exact reasons for the
benefits, they speculate that the bacteria used in fermenting
milk changes the bacteria already inside the stomach and
intestines. Those changes may help the body absorb nutrients
and produce enzymes needed for proper digestion of milk
proteins, among other functions.

Fermented milk is identified by the bacteria it contains,
and not all types are equally beneficial. Thermophilus milk,
for example, is effective in reducing lactose intolerance, but
buttermilk is not. Acidophilus milk has laxative effects in
older patients. It also has slowed growth of tumors in mice.
Other studies have shown that it eliminated some forms of

digestive tract infections.

Drinking fermented milk also helps to ease travelers' diarrhea.

Yogurt bacteria, injected directly into mouse tumors, made the growths shrink, the report says. Researchers believe that the bacteria stimulate the immune system into action, because the animals tested survived more than one bout with cancer.

Yogurt — probably the most popular form of fermented milk — also is a good source of protein, riboflavin (vitamin B2) and folic acid (one of the B-vitamin group).

A four-ounce serving has 115 calories, about one-half that of premium ice cream, and contains a teaspoon of fat. "Light" yogurt has fewer calories and less fat. Frozen yogurt has about the same amount of sugar, calcium, calories and protein as the equivalent amount of ice milk, but less fat.

For most folks, fermented milk like yogurt may be a good, natural way to raise overall immunity levels and fight some kinds of digestive problems.

## A cup of yogurt a day keeps the gynecologist away

Eating a cup of yogurt a day dramatically reduced recurring vaginitis in 11 women participating in a year-long study at the Long Island Jewish Medical Center in New York, according to a report in *Medical World News* (30,20:41).

Women suffering five or more episodes of vaginitis a year

were eligible for the study.

Simply eating yogurt was so beneficial that two dozen women refused to participate in the "no treatment" portion of the study.

"The number of infections fell from a mean of three to less than one during six months of daily yogurt consumption," according to the report.

Vaginitis is an infection of the female vagina, resulting in pain, burning and discomforting secretions.

Not all yogurt will work, however, researchers point out.

Only yogurt containing the bacteria Lactobacillus acidophilus is effective, but it is difficult to come by.

After testing various national brands, researchers say Columbo's was the only brand they found that contained L. acidophilus.

If women cannot find Columbo's yogurt in their grocery store, they "should consider making their own yogurt with acidophilus milk," these researchers suggest.


# The benefits of rice bran


Oat bran and wheat bran aren't the only bran you should be eating. New studies have shown that rice bran is more effective than wheat bran in providing bulk and protecting against colon cancer. Like oat bran, rice bran is also effective in lowering total cholesterol.

Rice bran is "nutritious, has a light, slightly sweet taste, is a good source of protein and iron, and yet is low in calories and sodium," says Doug Babcock in *Cereal Foods World* (32:8, 538). "Rice products are hypoallergenic and easily digestible." Rice is also cholesterol free and "contains only a trace of fat," explains Cornell University's *Consumer News*. "Rice is an excellent source of complex carbohydrates and provides thiamine, niacin, riboflavin, iron, calcium, fiber, phosphorus and protein," *Consumer News* continued.

"It has long been known that the bran layers of the rice kernel contain the highest concentration of nutrients," Babcock notes. "To gain the most food value, brown rice, which contains the bran layers, was the obvious choice. In fact, until recently, that was the only way we could enjoy the benefits of rice bran." Now stabilized rice bran is available separately and can be added to your daily diet.

Researchers at the Royal Hallamshire Hospital in Sheffield, England, recently compared rice bran and wheat bran. "The results of this study indicate that rice bran is an efficient stool bulking agent," said J. Tomlin, who led the research team for the report in *European Journal of Clinical Nutrition* (42:857). Even though volunteers only ate a slightly larger amount of rice bran, "it increased stool mass and frequency by over twice the increase caused by wheat bran."

The more bulk created in the stool and the faster the waste can be moved from the intestines, the lower the incidence of colon cancer. Rice bran is a type of dietary fiber, commonly known as roughage, that decreases the risk of colon cancer because it helps move waste products through the intestines rapidly. With less contact with the lining of the intestines, the cancer-causing contents in the intestines seem to be less harmful.

In a separate study in Japan reported in *Journal of Nutritional Science Vitaminology* (32:581), researchers compared a brown rice diet to a diet of polished rice, where the bran was removed. "The results suggest that rice fiber produced an increase in fecal weight, which is assumed to be effective in preventing colonic disease in advanced countries," the researchers concluded.

Your fiber intake should be at least 30 grams each day and include a variety of fiber types, according to the National Cancer Institute. "Dietitians recommend a high-fiber diet for patients with cardiovascular problems, obesity and diabetes, diverticulitis, and gastrointestinal problems or diseases," according to Babcock.

Another benefit of rice bran is that it can lower levels of total cholesterol, low density lipoprotein (LDL) and very low density lipoprotein, while raising the amount of high density lipoprotein (HDL), according to a study in *Lipids* (21:715). Low density lipoproteins are the dangerous type of cholesterol that increases the risk of heart disease. High density lipoprotein, sometimes called the "good" cholesterol, helps protect the body against heart and artery disease.

Other research at the U.S. Department of Agriculture (USDA) in Albany, California, shows that rice bran lowers total cholesterol as well as oat bran, reports *Science News* (134:20, 308). "Preliminary results show a balanced diet, including 10 percent dietary fiber from defatted rice bran, reduces cholesterol in hamsters by more than 25 percent."

In diabetics, rice helped lower cholesterol levels when it replaced potatoes. "When rice was the major carbohydrate source the very low density lipoprotein triglycerides decreased," the *American Journal of Clinical Nutrition* (39:598) reported.

Lowering blood cholesterol levels is important because it can reduce the rate of coronary heart disease and hardening of the arteries. As early as 1947, a study of heart disease in seven nations showed a direct relationship between a country's incidence of heart disease, the level of cholesterol in the blood and the amount of animal fat in the national diet.

A third major benefit of rice bran is that it helps lower the incidence of calcium-containing urinary stones by decreasing the amount of calcium excreted in the urine, reports the *Journal of Urology* (132:1140). "In almost all patients, rice bran caused a significant decrease in urinary calcium excretion," wrote Dr. Ohkawa, one of the researchers. "Evidence of stones has decreased clearly among patients treated with rice bran for one to three years ... We suggest that ... rice bran treatment should be effective for prevention of recurrent urinary stone disease."

The *British Journal of Urology* (58:592) has also reported rice bran's ability to limit urinary calcium and stone production.

## Use moderation in eating oat bran

He must have thought, if a little oat bran is good, a lot is better. That's why a 75-year-old man ended up in a Connecticut hospital with nausea, abdominal pain, frequent vomiting and a week without bowel movements, according to a report in *The New England Journal of Medicine* (320,17:1148).

Surgeons opened up his lower intestine and found a 2-foot-long plug of "vegetable matter" that completely blocked his small bowel. They removed the mass, and three weeks later the man went home. Doctors discovered that a week before he had to check into the hospital, the man had begun eating 60 grams (a little over two ounces) a day of oat bran in the form of oat bran muffins.

Six years before that, the man had part of his intestine removed because of diverticulitis. Some inside scars from that operation, along with the "excessively high dose" of oat bran and the suddenness of the high dose without any gradual increase, probably caused the man's problem, the doctors speculate.

"We suggest that caution be exercised in the prescription of large doses of bran for the patient who has had abdominal surgery," the doctors advise. A daily maximum intake of between 10 to 25 grams (under a half-ounce up to just under one ounce) would be better, the report says. There should also be a gradual "breaking-in" period, starting with low doses of bran, before building up to the maximum, the doctors say.

## Some herbal teas are toxic

If you enjoy brewing herbal teas, or even growing and mixing your own, take note. Some herbal teas, especially those that are home-grown, are toxic and can lead to liver, digestive and nervous-system disorders, according to a report in *American Family Physician* (39,5:153).

"Most commercial herbal teas are considered safe," says Dr. Paul M. Ridker, author of the report. But "Lewis Carroll's account of Alice's tea party, during which the participants became 'mad as a hatter' and 'dry as a bone,' aptly describes the effects of some herbal teas," says the doctor.

Herbal remedies were widely used by 19th-century physicians to treat a host of ailments. As modern medicine developed, "folkloric" remedies fell by the wayside, although the public's interest in herbs did not. Understandably, today's physicians are not as well versed in herbal toxicities, but they are catching up, Dr. Ridker says.

Many people enjoy growing their own herbs for teas and cooking, and for the most part, herbs are safe to use. But mark the following herbal teas as potentially dangerous and possibly unsafe to drink:

- **Comfrey, groundsel, gordolobo, sassafras, T'u-San-Chi and tansy ragwort** — These teas have sometimes caused liver failure, which is "among the most worrisome complications of herbal tea exposure," according to Dr. Ridker.

The danger of comfrey tea is confirmed in a report in *The Lancet* (1,8639:657), a research journal published in both the U.S. and England. Teas made from the comfrey plant have been marketed in many countries in the past as "natural" remedies for everything from arthritis to infections. At least four different toxic alkaloids have been identified in common comfrey, prickly comfrey and

Russian comfrey. The poisons attack the liver, sometimes causing hepatic veno-occlusive disease, a form of worsening portal hypertension. Portal hypertension is a kind of high blood pressure involving the liver, and can lead to liver failure and death. In addition, the comfrey poisons are linked to higher rates of cancer and lung tumors in animal tests.

"Comfrey products are marketed as herbal teas, herb root powders, and as capsules: their continued availability must be questioned," the report warned. Canada already has attempted to ban the sale of some comfrey products. The report concluded that the number of comfrey tea-related poisonings may be "grossly underestimated."

• **Senna, pokeroot and buckthorn** — These teas may cause diarrhea, hypotension (low blood pressure) and dehydration.

• **Lobelia, burdock, thorn apple and jimson weed** — These teas may cause delirium, disorientation, blurred vision, dry mouth and dilated pupils.

• **Melilot, woodruff and tonka bean** — These teas contain coumarin, which causes an anticoagulant (anti-clotting) effect, and are especially dangerous for people already taking anticoagulant medication or large doses of aspirin.

Another problem is contamination of some otherwise harmless teas with dangerous additional plants. Researchers have identified foxglove, squill, lily of the valley, yellow oleander and common oleander as contaminates of some herbal teas.

These substances may mimic the effects of cardiac glycosides, which are found in heart-stimulating medications such as digitalis (which, incidentally, is another name for foxglove). On the other hand, mint, raspberry, blackberry, rose hips and citrus peel teas are beneficial and are *not* harmful.

According to Dr. Ridker, "Labels warning of potentially dangerous side effects of tea constituents are currently not required, and inadvertent exposure to toxic ingredients in herbal teas is likely to continue."

The Canadian Health Protection Branch (similar to the U.S. Food and Drug Administration) began regulating herbs in March 1989, and controversy has been brewing ever since, according to *Herbalgram* (20:14). The Canadian agency singled out herbs because they are not a food and not a drug. They fall somewhere in between and were not previously regulated.

The regulations divide plants into two classifications. On the first list, the HPB identified herbs that cannot be sold as food; in effect, they are banned substances. The second list identified herbs that must be sold with labels warning about toxicity.

Opponents charge that the HPB has not been consistent in regulating foods used for medicinal purposes. Prunes, for example, are known for their laxative effects but are not regulated, and coffee does not have labels cautioning consumers about its diuretic effects.

The HPB may have bitten off more than it can chew in trying to regulate foods that contain carcinogens, cancer-causing agents. Opponents argue that "99 percent of the known carcinogens are of natural origin." To date, sassafras is the only carcinogen-containing plant that is banned in Canada.

# Vegetable variety a key to preventing lung cancer

To lower your risk of lung cancer, you should eat a variety of fruits and vegetables, such as tomatoes, broccoli and cabbage, researchers report in *Science News* (136,7:102) and the *Journal of the National Cancer Institute* (81,15:1158). Researchers say those foods contain substances that prevent tumor growth and can reduce your lung-cancer risk — even if you smoke.

In the study, females got big benefits from a wide variety of vegetables. Women registered a cancer risk decrease of seven-fold, while men were "only" three times less likely to get lung cancer by eating lots of different veggies, the *SN* report says. Women seemed to benefit slightly more from a single substance, beta-carotene, than men. Women had a three-fold risk reduction, compared to two-fold for men.

Previous lung-cancer research centered on the anticancer properties of beta-carotene, a component of vitamin A found in carrots, papaya, mangoes, sweet potatoes and some other vegetables. But researchers have discovered that other substances related to beta-carotene—lutein, indoles and lycopene — seem to be just as beneficial.

Lutein is found in watercress, spinach, broccoli, green pepper and other dark green vegetables. Broccoli also contains indoles. Researchers have known for some time that broccoli and cabbage, known as cruciferous vegetables, also help prevent colon cancer. Tomatoes (including tomato juice) contain lycopene and are the only fruit shown to have the same beneficial properties as vegetables, researchers say.

Researchers say eating a variety of vegetables is good for smokers as well. In their study of 230 men and 102 women with lung cancer and 597 men and 268 women controls, researchers found the greatest risk reduction among men who were heavy smokers or recent ex-smokers and women who were light smokers.

## Fish oil as a natural healer

An increasing number of researchers and physicians are discovering the many healing benefits of a natural ingredient called omega-3 fatty acids by scientists and simply "fish oil" by the rest of us. Population studies show that people who eat substantial amounts of cold-water fish have lower rates of coronary artery disease than other people, even if the total amounts of fat in the diets of both groups is about the same. Recent studies suggest that the addition of fish to the diet, especially replacing red meat and dairy products with fish, will have a positive health benefit.

Norwegian researchers, led by Kristian Bjerve, discovered that omega-3 fatty acids are essential for the normal metabolic processing of another kind of dietary oil, omega-6 fatty acids. Omega-6 oils are close relatives of omega-3 oils and are found in things like safflower oil and other cooking oils.

The Norwegians found a direct relationship between daily doses of omega-3 oils and healthy levels of certain blood substances. In their study, they found that 350 to 400 milligrams of omega-3 acids in the form of purified fish oil are needed daily to maintain normal plasma and lipid levels. "Omega-3 fatty acids possibly also have some specific function in the retina (in the eye) and in the central nervous system," Bjerve says.

"Dietary fish oils are rich in eicosapentaenoic acid (EPA), a polyunsaturated fatty acid of the omega-3 series," according to *Postgraduate Medicine* (85,4: 406). Essential fatty acids, like EPA, have been discovered to play important roles "in the control and prevention" of heart and artery disease, the lowering of high blood pressure and preventing unnecessary blood clotting.

Current research is also investigating fish oil's potential to help in angina (heart pain), rheumatoid arthritis and other inflammatory disorders, kidney disease and breast cancer, *Postgraduate Medicine* reports.

Another study at the Pennington Biomedical Research Center in Baton Rouge, La., found that fish oil's anti-clotting action in animals "depends on the dosage of fish oil *in relation* to other kinds of polyunsaturated fats — not the absolute amount of fish oil consumed," *Science News* (135,12:183) reports.

"If confirmed in humans, the finding may lead to recommendations on how much of the different kinds of polyunsaturated fats people should consume," says the *Science News* report. Since a daily requirement has not been set, and safe levels of fish oil supplements have not been established, "the consumption of fresh fish two to three times weekly is likely a reasonable recommendation," says the *Postgraduate Medicine* report.

Here are some ways that fish oil helps to prevent artery disease:

• **Provides healing inside blood vessels.** The insides of arteries suffer injuries, sometimes from turbulent blood flow. Sticky platelets in the blood collect around the injured area and send chemical signals for more sticky helpers, including germ-fighting white cells. The result, sometimes, is too much help.

Cholesterol, a natural part of blood, collects in unusual amounts at the growing bottleneck in the busy blood pipeline. The "helpers" continue to send signals that cause more of the blood's clotting agents to pile on the growing mass. The result is atherosclerosis: a form of hardening of the arteries caused by fatty plaque growing on and changing the walls inside arteries.

These plaque blockages reduce blood flow, especially in arteries feeding the heart. Reduced blood flow, in turn, starves whole areas of heart muscle, resulting in heart pain (angina) or even heart attacks. Plaque blockages also cause blood clots to form, further reducing blood flow. That can happen in many areas of the body besides the heart.

Omega-3 fish oil helps the healing process by making the blood helpers less sticky, and by keeping them from piling up and blocking the artery.

• **Fortifies cells.** One part of the fish oil, EPA (eicosapentaenoic acid), gets into the cells that make up the artery walls. The EPA-fortified cells start cranking out their own chemical signals that order sticky, clot-forming platelets to stay away.

"Increasing fish oil in the diet leads to a slight lowering of cholesterol (of the harmful LDL type), and it sometimes reduces high blood pressure as well," reports Dr. Alexander Leaf, writing in *Your Good Health,* a publication of Harvard Medical School.

Other studies reported in *Total Nutrition Guide* (Bantam Books, pg. 43) suggest it helps the joints, cuts down on arthritis discomfort, and reduces the pain of and even prevents migraine headaches.

More recent animal studies reported in *Science News* (134:228) indicate that well-fed mice on high-fat diets that included fish oils rich in omega-3 displayed the following responses:

(1) lived twice as long as normal mice;

(2) had half the normal levels of harmful autoimmune responses (inflammatory diseases like rheumatoid arthritis and lupus, in which antibodies attack the body's own tissues);

(3) showed a complete absence of kidney disease, which normally strikes all these kinds of test animals; and

(4) had blood cholesterol levels half that in normal mice, even lower than those in another study group of mice that had been fed calorie-restricted, low-fat diets.

Researchers are now testing fish oil in people to see what effect it has under clinical conditions on several other diseases. These problems being researched include psoriasis, nephritis (inflammation of the kidneys), lupus, arthritis, and some forms of cancers involving the immune system.

Although you can get fish oil supplements (usually sold as omega-3 in capsule form), many physicians say a safer way is to forget the pills and eat fish containing the oils. To get adequate amounts of omega-3 acids, fish oil supplements must be taken in high doses, which can cause several problems, including:

- Diarrhea, flatulence (gas) and upset stomach.
- Reducing the blood's ability to clot. Increased bleeding time could be very dangerous and in some cases could cause fatal hemorrhaging, reports *The Medical Letter* (29:731). Anyone taking blood thinning drugs or aspirin therapy, who is planning surgery, or who has a family history of strokes or hemorrhaging should avoid fish oil supplements.
- Consuming high amounts of vitamin E. Large doses of fish oil supplements could cause someone to ingest large amounts of vitamin E. In large doses, vitamin E hinders the blood's ability to clot (which adds to the above-mentioned problems) and can cause possibly fatal results, according to a study by Pauling and Enstrom.
- Raising blood sugar levels in diabetics. People with

inactive diabetes may discover that the fish oil activates their diabetes, says Harry S. Glauber of the University of California at San Diego. Jan Lipkin of the American Diabetes Association says use of fish oil supplements "makes it harder for patients to control their blood sugar levels." Glauber and the American Diabetes Association recommend that diabetics and people at high risk for developing diabetes should avoid fish oil supplements.

- High amounts of vitamin A, which can be toxic, reports the *New England Journal of Medicine* (316: 10, 626).
- Toxic amounts of vitamin D, reports the American Diabetes Association.
- Cod liver oil should be avoided because it contains cholesterol and can lead to overdoses of vitamins A and D, according to Dr. Nathaniel Shafer of New York Medical College in *The Medical Tribune*.

The highest levels of the two kinds of beneficial fish oil ingredients (EPA and DHA fatty acids) are found in fresh or frozen fish that normally live in deep, cold waters. Eating canned fish is not recommended, since the canning process destroys most of the omega-3 oil.

The best of the saltwater breeds are mackerel (Atlantic, king and chub), Pacific and Atlantic herring, European anchovies, chinook salmon, sablefish, sturgeon, tuna and mullet. Cod is a cold-water fish, but has relatively little omega-3 oil in its flesh. Instead, the cod stores omega-3 in its liver. But many doctors advise against a regular supplement of cod liver oil, since too much of the old remedy can cause overdoses of vitamins A, D and E.

Among freshwater fish, highest omega-3 levels are found in lake trout and whitefish. Shellfish like lobster, crab and shrimp have smaller amounts of omega-3, as do mollusks like scallops and clams.

If you don't like fish that much, you can still get some EPA through plant sources, according to *Everyday Health Tips* (Rodale Press, pg. 74). But, most plants generally are lower in omega-3 than the same amounts of fish. However, there are exceptions. For example, oat germ is a good source of omega-3, better than all but 15 kinds of oil-rich fish. Three and one-half ounces of oat germ has more omega-3 than the same amount of sockeye salmon or mullet.

Common dry beans have more omega-3 than ocean perch, Pacific halibut, red snapper and many other kinds of fish. The lettuce-like purslane, used in soups and salads in Mediterranean countries, is high in EPA. Also good are tofu, walnuts, wheat germ oil, several kinds of beans, soybean products and rapeseed oil.

Margarine also is a rich source of omega-3, largely because it's made from soybeans. Unfortunately, it also has more saturated fats than fish or other plant sources of omega-3.

Some people shouldn't take fish oil supplements or eat higher than normal amounts of food containing EPA and DHA.

Those with diabetes, persons with a history of hemorrhaging or strokes, or patients facing surgery or on aspirin and blood-thinning therapy should avoid fish oil unless specifically authorized by their doctors.

# Fish oil's top 20

Based on an uncooked serving size of 100 grams (approximately three and one-half ounces), the following kinds of fish are highest in total omega-3 fatty acids content.

| Fish | Total Fat | Omega-3 |
|------|-----------|---------|
| Atlantic mackerel | 13.9 | 2.6 |
| Chub mackerel | 11.5 | 2.2 |
| King mackerel | 13.0 | 2.2 |
| Lake trout | 9.7 | 2.0 |
| Japanese horse mackerel | 7.8 | 1.9 |
| Pacific herring | 13.9 | 1.8 |
| Atlantic herring | 9.0 | 1.7 |
| Bluefin tuna | 6.6 | 1.6 |
| Albacore tuna | 4.9 | 1.5 |
| Sablefish | 15.3 | 1.5 |
| Chinook salmon | 10.4 | 1.5 |
| Atlantic sturgeon | 6.0 | 1.5 |
| Lake whitefish | 6.0 | 1.5 |
| European anchovy | 4.8 | 1.4 |
| Atlantic salmon | 5.4 | 1.4 |
| Round herring | 4.4 | 1.3 |
| Sockeye salmon | 8.6 | 1.3 |
| Sprat | 5.8 | 1.3 |
| Bluefish | 6.5 | 1.2 |
| Mullet | 4.4 | 1.1 |

SOURCE — U.S. Department of Agriculture, Human
Nutrition Information Service

# Best plant sources of omega-3

The following are plant sources high in omega-3 fatty
acids. The comparisons are based on a serving size of approximately three and one-half ounces (100 grams).

| Food | Total fat (in grams) | Total cholesterol | Total omega-3 |
|---|---|---|---|
| Rapeseed oil | 100 | 0 | 11.1 |
| Walnut oil | 100 | 0 | 10.4 |
| Wheat germ oil | 100 | 0 | 6.9 |
| Soybean oil | 100 | 0 | 6.8 |
| English walnuts | 61.9 | 0 | 6.8 |
| Black walnuts | 56.6 | 0 | 3.3 |
| Tomato seed oil | 100 | 0 | 2.3 |
| Soybeans, sprouted, cooked | 4.5 | 0 | 2.1 |
| Dry soybeans | 21.3 | 0 | 1.6 |
| Oat germ | 30.7 | 0 | 1.4 |
| Leeks, raw | 2.1 | 0 | 0.7 |
| Radish seeds, sprouted | 2.5 | 0 | 0.7 |
| Wheat germ | 10.9 | 0 | 0.7 |
| Common dry beans | 1.5 | 0 | 0.6 |
| Navy beans | 0.8 | 0 | 0.3 |
| Pinto beans | 0.9 | 0 | 0.3 |

## Other sources (for comparison)

| Food | Total fat (grams) | Total cholesterol | Total omega-3 |
|---|---|---|---|
| Salad dressing, blue cheese, commercial | 52.3 | 17 | 3.7 |
| Salad dressing, Italian, commercial brands | 48.3 | 0 | 3.3 |
| Hard margarine, made with soybean | 80.5 | 0 | 3.0 |
| Butter | 81.1 | 2.19 | 1.2 |
| Shortening, household lard and vegetable oil | 100 | 56 | 1.1 |
| Cured pork bacon, raw | 57.5 | 67 | 0.8 |
| Fresh pork, trimmed | 76.7 | 93 | 0.7 |
| Whole milk | 3.3 | 14 | 0.1 |
| Chicken, white meat, no skin | 1.7 | 58 | trace |

SOURCE: U.S. Department of Agriculture, Human Nutrition Information Service

## Danger from a Japanese dish

Doctors operating on the 24-year-old college student thought the patient had appendicitis. He had been hospitalized with pain and tenderness in the lower right part of his abdomen. But when they opened him up, they found everything normal and healthy.

Normal, that is, until the surgeon — about to sew up the incision — was shocked to see a bright red worm an inch and a half long crawl out of the man's intestinal cavity onto a surgical cloth near the wound. The patient recovered nicely, but the worm died, doctors report in *The New England Journal of Medicine* (320,17:1124).

It turns out the young man had eaten a dish that's become popular in this country recently — sushi, a meal of raw fish long associated with Japan. He ate it the night before at a friend's house, according to an Associated Press report.

Cooking would kill any fish parasites like the eustrongylides, the worm found in the man's innards. But since some oriental fish dishes like sushi and sashimi are normally served raw or nearly raw, some internal fish parasites may come along for a live ride into a human digestive tract.

Once inside, such nematodes and other parasites can live long enough to cause severe lower abdominal pain. Occasionally, some worms can pierce the digestive tract and enter into the peritoneal cavity, causing more serious problems, including the risk of infection.

The report says that such parasites can show up in both salt and freshwater fish. Commercial fish that may be infected include mackerel, herring, rockfish, salmon and cod. Pacific fish are more likely to have the parasites than Atlantic catches.

Avoid the problem by fully cooking all fish that you eat, the journal recommends.

## For health's sake, take coarse approach to baking

Using coarse flour for routine baking may lower your risk of getting high blood pressure, hardening of the arteries, gallstones, obesity and diseases of the colon, even colon cancer, a new report says. That's the suggestion from three doctors at the Bristol Royal Infirmary in England, as reported in *British Medical Journal* (298,6688:1616).

Part of the healthful effect of coarsely ground flour may be because it escapes complete digestion in the stomach and upper intestines, the doctors say. "Overefficient digestion of starch" may give rise to excess levels of insulin in the blood and to problems with the colon, the lower end of the digestive tract, the report suggests. Some doctors think that some cases of high blood pressure may be triggered by problems with insulin levels.

Undigested coarse flour also could beneficially affect the colon like rough dietary fiber, the doctors say. For those reasons, they tested the theory on 20 patients who either suffered from non-insulin-dependent diabetes or had undergone colon surgery to treat ulcerative colitis.

"In both groups, the meal containing bread made from coarse flour resulted in lower plasma glucose and insulin concentrations than that containing bread made from fine flour," the report says. "Thus the risk of some colonic diseases, including cancer, might be reduced if coarse flour was eaten regularly and combined with other less completely digested starchy foods," the doctors conclude.

The researchers also suggest that diabetics may achieve better control of blood sugar levels by eating breads baked from coarse flour.

Here's how the doctors measure whether flour is coarse: nearly half the flour won't pass through a sieve with holes one millimeter wide, and at least 80 percent of the flour won't pass through holes of 140 micrometers diameter.

## New sweetener approved

A calorie-free sweetener that can be used in cooking has just been approved by the U.S. Food and Drug Administration (F.D.A.).

Sunette®, technically known as acesulfame K, may provide new options for weight-conscious people because it can tolerate high temperatures. The popular sweetener aspertame (Nutra Sweet®) breaks down at high temperatures and cannot be used in baked goods.

The F.D.A. approved Sunette® for use in several dry foods, including pudding mixes, sweetener packets, and chewing gum.

## Don't poison yourself with potatoes

Beware of eating potatoes that have shriveled brown spots on the skins. Store-bought potatoes with these signs of potato dry-rot may contain harmful levels of a poison produced by a plant fungus, according to a biochemist with the federal government.

Potato poisoning, even at low levels from only one or two potatoes, can cause vomiting, hair loss, a damaged immune system, nervous system problems, coma and even death, according to Anne E. Desjardins of the U.S. Department of Agriculture's Research Service in Peoria, Ill.

The finding of danger from potato fungus poisoning is new, she says in *Science News* (135,15:238). One other study in France also showed dangerous levels of the poison trichothecenes in some ordinary potatoes bought in grocery stores there.

Just cutting off the obvious rotted part of the potato won't remove all the poison, the researcher says. Even disease-free parts of those potatoes studied contained about 10 percent of the amount of poison found in the rotted parts, says Desjardins. That's still enough to cause sickness.

Another danger — the fungus-produced poison is heat-stable, meaning that normal cooking methods won't remove or lessen the danger.

# Premenstrual Syndrome (PMS)

## Relief from PMS

The monthly terrors of PMS (premenstrual syndrome) can be relieved with these suggestions:

- Vitamin B6 (pyridoxine) should be taken daily in premenstrual times. It helps relieve fluid retention, weight gain, arthritis associated with female hormone deficiency, and symptoms of depression.
- Supplements of the amino acid DLPA (d,l, phenylalanine) provide amazing relief to chronic PMS sufferers, according to current research. This amino acid has been found to be the substance in chocolate that causes many people to crave chocolate. For maximum effectiveness, supplements should be taken daily at mealtimes for several weeks.

- Avoid coffee and caffeine. The more coffee you drink, the more severe your PMS symptoms usually become says a report in the *American Journal of Public Health* (75,11:1135). Women with the most severe PMS problems were found to drink four or more cups of coffee daily. Despite this discovery, many over-the-counter products for PMS contain caffeine. So remember to read the labels.

# Sleeping Problems

## A medical reason for your tiredness

If you are tired in the morning and sleepy throughout the day, you might be suffering from sleep apnea (pronounced **ap-nee-a**). Apnea is a medical problem that causes people to stop breathing at least five times during the night for periods of 20 to 40 seconds each time. These stoppages decrease the supply of oxygen to the brain, resulting in sleepiness and loss of concentration during waking hours, especially in the evening.

Typical sufferers are men who are loud snorers, overweight, and are middle-aged or elderly, says a report from the American Lung Association. Many also suffer, knowingly or not, from high blood pressure.

Sleep apnea presents an even greater problem for people who drive, such as truck drivers. Researchers at a sleep-disorder clinic report that the auto-accident rate for people with severe sleep apnea is seven times that of the normal population and accounts for 38,000 accidents per year in the United States says a report in the *American Review of Respiratory Disease* (August 1989). Even minor, easily controlled sleep disturbances can impair driving ability. But many people fail to tell their doctors about the problem because they fear losing their drivers' licenses.

Perhaps the most common cause of sleep apnea is being fat. Obesity causes an excessive amount of soft tissue to accumulate in the throat, resulting in an obstructed airway, snoring and apnea. You can help treat the underlying cause of your sleeping disorder by losing weight and quitting smoking, says a report in *British Medical Journal* (298, 6678:904).

The most annoying symptom of apnea — for people who live with you, that is — is snoring. To fight snoring, try propping your head up at night. Or, if you snore only while lying on your back, sew a tennis ball into the back of your pajama top. That will prompt you to roll over onto your side or stomach.

Finally, if you think your problem is beyond your control, see your doctor, who can bring you up-to-date on the latest medical techniques to treat sleeping disorders. Surgery to correct apnea is a last resort. If you have a sleep disorder and your physican has advised you not to drive until your condition is controlled, take the advice. If you don't and are involved in an accident, your insurance company may claim that you were driving against medical advice.

# Strokes

## Know the warning signs of stroke

If you had a sudden pain in your chest, you'd probably recognize it as a possible warning of a heart attack.

But what if one arm or leg suddenly becomes weak or numb? Or without warning, you get dizzy, have double vision or lose sight in one eye? You have difficulty speaking, standing or walking. Would you recognize these seemingly unrelated problems as warning signs for stroke, the third leading cause of death and a major source of disability?

About 10 percent of strokes are preceded by "transient ischemic attacks" or TIAs, the American Heart Association (AHA) reports. TIAs are sometimes called "little strokes" because the symptoms affect limbs, vision, balance or speech and last only for a few minutes. But TIAs can precede a stroke and should be considered a warning, says the AHA. People who have experienced one of these temporary blockages of blood flow to some part of the brain are nearly 10 times more likely to suffer a paralyzing stroke than those who haven't had a TIA.

"It's important for the public to realize that the symptoms, or warning signs, for stroke are diverse," points out Dr. Louis R. Caplan of Boston, chairperson of the AHA Stroke Council. "They're not as clear-cut as heart attack symptoms."

The problem is that most people don't understand how the brain works, says Caplan. "So when these warning signs strike, they don't link it to the nervous system. Prompt medical or surgical attention to these warning signs can prevent a fatal or disabling stroke from occurring."

Since 38 percent of all stroke victims die within a month, the 30 days following a stroke are critical. Yet nearly half the people who survive the first month are still living seven years after their stroke, the AHA discovered. So although a stroke is serious, quick medical attention can make an important difference in its effects.

Anyone at high risk for having a stroke should try to lower the risk by reducing or eliminating some of the factors that can be controlled. High blood pressure, heart disease, high red blood cell count, transient ischemic attacks (TIAs), elevated blood cholesterol, cigarette smoking, excessive alcohol intake, physical inactivity and obesity are factors that increase the risk of stroke — but these factors can be treated or eliminated. You can quit smoking, lower your blood pressure, increase your physical activity and lose weight to help lower your risk of stroke.

There are also several risk factors which cannot be changed — age, sex, race, diabetes mellitus, prior stroke, heredity, and "asymptomatic carotid bruit" (a bruit indicates a blockage that may be reducing blood flow to the brain). People with several of stroke's risk factors should be especially careful to know and watch for stroke's warning signals.

In summary, here are the major warning signals of stroke:

• sudden weakness or numbness of the face, arm and leg on one side of the body
• loss of speech, or trouble talking or understanding speech
• dimness or loss of vision, particularly in only one eye
• unexplained dizziness, especially when associated with other neurological symptoms
• unusual and severe headaches
• any paralysis on one side of the body.

If you experience any of these symptoms, call your doctor and get medical help.

## More strokes diagnosed, but fewer deaths occur

More people are diagnosed with stroke but fewer are dying from strokes, a 30-year study in Framingham, Mass., reveals.

Even though there has been a dramatic increase in the number of strokes in the United States, especially in men, the American Heart Association (AHA) reports that the death rate from stroke has fallen dramatically during the second half of this century. In 1950, 88.8 of every 100,000 Americans died of a stroke; by 1985 it had been reduced to 32.8 deaths per 100,000.

The doctors are not sure why the death rate fell. "Our hunch is that it is due to either a decline in the severity of the stroke or better detection. We are perhaps able now to detect more mild cases," said Boston University neurologist Dr. Philip A. Wolf.

Better detection includes new diagnostic techniques that enable doctors to discover mild strokes that could not be detected just 10 years ago. One of the most important diagnostic tools is the computerized tomography (CT) brain scan which can confirm a stroke much earlier and with fewer noticeable symptoms than in the past.

In the study led by Wolfe, researchers looked at stroke incidence and death rates in men and women, aged 55 to 64, from 1953 to 1983. "When we looked at the incidence, we found that people with stroke are less likely to die even though there have not been any dramatic breakthroughs with stroke, such as there has been for coronary artery disease with coronary care units," Wolf reports.

The decline in stroke death rates is not confined to the Framingham study. Results of a Rochester, Minn., survey suggest that the decreasing stroke death rate may be due to better detection and control of high blood pressure.

In most Western countries this extraordinary phenomenon has been going on for 20 years or more, with an over 50 percent decline being recorded in death rates from stroke, the AHA reports. "Without any doubt," Wolf says, "there seems to be a substantial and significant decline in death rates from stroke."

Despite an average 5.5 percent annual decline since 1973, stroke afflicts approximately half a million Americans each year, according to the AHA. Stroke claimed more than 147,800 lives in 1986, the most recent year for which statistics are available. Stroke is the nation's third-ranking killer, after heart attack and cancer.

## Low cholesterol linked to strokes in some men

A man who has a combination of high blood pressure and low levels of total cholesterol may face an increased risk of death from a bleeding stroke, according to a new research report. But the researchers warn that low cholesterol levels are still desirable for most people because the risk of death from heart and artery disease, or from a nonbleeding stroke, is much greater than the risk from a bleeding stroke.

For bleeding strokes, known as hemorrhagic strokes, "the death rate was highest in the lower cholesterol category (less than 160 milligrams of cholesterol per deciliter of blood volume) and decreased with increasing cholesterol levels," according to the report in the *New England Journal of Medicine* (320,14:904).

The researchers suggest that very low serum cholesterol levels cause an increase in strokes. That's because low cholesterol seems to result in weakened walls of arteries in the brain. Just as water under pressure seeks a weak spot in a hose to burst through, high blood pressure increases the strain on the arteries and increases the number of ruptures or bleeding strokes, they believe.

However, high levels of cholesterol are known to cause an increased risk of death due to heart or artery disease, or due to nonbleeding strokes. "Within every cholesterol-level category, age-adjusted death rates for coronary heart disease were higher than for all strokes." In this study, 60.5 men out of 10,000 died of coronary heart disease compared to just 2.36 who died from a bleeding stroke.

According to the American Heart Association, about 10 percent of all strokes result from cerebral hemorrhages, when a defective artery in the brain bursts, flooding the surrounding tissue with blood. The loss of a constant supply of blood means that some brain cells no longer can function. The accumulated blood from the burst artery may put pressure on surrounding brain tissue and interfere with the way the brain operates.

"The men who died from each type of stroke were older, had higher systolic and diastolic blood pressure, were more likely to smoke cigarettes, and were more likely to be black," the researchers noted.

The study seems to indicate that for a few men, the danger of having a bleeding stroke may be high enough to warrant an increased risk of other kinds of diseases caused by high cholesterol levels. That can be determined only after medical testing and talking with a doctor.

But for most people, lowering blood cholesterol is still a healthy target.

# The nutrient that cuts the risk of fatal stroke by nearly half

There's an easy way to slash your risk of having a fatal stroke — eat one extra serving of fresh fruit or vegetables every day, declares a major new dietary study.

The super stroke preventer is the nutrient potassium, abundant in fresh fruits and vegetables, according to doctors Kay-Tee Khaw and Elizabeth Barrett-Connor and reported in *Medical World News* (30,11:30).

These researchers raised the possibility of potassium being a stroke fighter in a big study in 1987. Since then, three separate medical studies have demonstrated that increased potassium in the diet can dramatically lower your risk of death from stroke, the report says.

The studies found that groups of people that ate the most fruits and vegetables had 25 to 40 percent fewer fatal strokes than groups with lower potassium intakes.

According to the report, women benefitted from a high potassium diet even more than men. The people in the studies all were 59 or older.

"Americans could raise their potassium levels significantly by simply cutting down on junk food and substituting orange or grapefruit juice for soft drinks," according to the report.

# Aspirin for stroke victims

An aspirin a day may be effective in preventing or reducing the effects of mental deterioration or dementia due to strokes.

Approximately 50 percent of dementia in elderly patients is related to Alzheimer's disease. However, the number two cause is dementia due to multiple strokes, known as MID (multi-infarct dementia). According to Dr. John S. Mery, of Baylor College of Medicine, Houston, about one-third of all dementia cases are caused by MID.

In a recent study, daily aspirin seemed to provide drastic improvements in MID patients. The researchers studied two groups of patients, whose average age was 67 years, with similar risk factors for stroke. They were treated identically, except that one group was given a single tablet of aspirin (325 milligrams) daily.

Blood flow in the brain and mental function improved significantly in the aspirin-treated patients, compared to the no-aspirin control group. The aspirin group also suffered fewer strokes or TIAs (transient ischemic attacks) than the no-aspirin group. "In the control group, 24 percent had subsequent strokes, while only 8.1 percent of the aspirin patients had strokes during the trial," Meyers said. TIAs occurred in 39.4 percent of the control patients, compared to just 18.9 of the patients treated with aspirin. A TIA is a temporary interference with the blood supply to the brain.

"We haven't found a cure for Alzheimer's yet, but we've got something (aspirin therapy) that is helping MID," Meyer explained. "That's why it is important to identify the cause of the dementia and treat the two groups of patients separately."

## Early warning sign for impending strokes — the eyes have it

Permanent blindness is one of the most feared of all disabilities, according to several polls taken in the United States.

As bad as blindness may be, a particular kind of temporary blindness may be a warning sign of something even worse — a stroke that might be fatal unless successful steps are taken to prevent it.

Persons over age 45 who experience a sudden loss of vision, lasting only a day or less, may be as much as 16 times more likely than the average person to suffer a massive, even fatal, stroke within a few weeks or months. That's the finding of British researchers reported in *The Lancet* (1,8631:185).

Medically, such an attack of temporary blindness is called lone bilateral blindness. The researchers are saying such attacks ought to be classified as telltale "preliminary" strokes that give advance signals of more life-threatening incidents soon to occur.

Here are the symptoms of this warning signal:

• A rapid dimming or complete loss of vision in both eyes at the same time
• The blindness lasts 24 hours or less

• More or less normal vision returns after no more than one day.

This particular temporary loss of vision occurs without any loss of consciousness, without any kind of seizure, and without any accompanying paralysis, dizziness or double vision. These symptoms distinguish this type of temporary blindness from some other types of vision problems.

Other kinds of temporary ("transient") blindness can occur during and after epileptic seizures, after childbirth, during heart attacks, after general anesthesia, as a result of brain tumors, and even during severe migraine headache attacks, the report says. However, these other kinds of temporary blindness are not advance signals of life-threatening strokes, according to the researchers. For five years, the researchers kept track of 14 patients who had experienced all the symptoms of lone bilateral blindness. The tracking was part of a larger study that followed 512 patients who had experienced transient ischemic attacks (TIA).

A TIA is what we would call a minor stroke, in which the stroke symptoms last for less than one day. A TIA generally is thought to be caused by high blood pressure-related problems, by blood clots in or near the brain, or by advanced diabetes.

Most of the 14 individuals said their loss of vision was either instantaneous or reached its maximum within seconds. Most said they experienced complete blindness very suddenly, but four patients "described their vision as dimming, frosting, or like looking through a haze or mist."

In all 14, the vision "loss was severe enough to make

reading or recognition of faces impossible and most were unable to see well enough to get about." Five of the 14 also said a headache accompanied the attack of blindness. Several reported sweating, buzzing in the head and chest discomfort during the attack.

Of the 14 patients with lone bilateral blindness, five suffered their first-ever stroke within two-and-a-half years. Statistically, that's about 16 times the number of strokes that would be expected in that same age group (average age 67 years) among the general population, the report says.

The researchers recommend that patients who have experienced attacks of lone bilateral blindness be considered high risks for stroke. They should be treated just like patients with diagnosed TIA — "by control of vascular risk factors and ... prophylactic aspirin."

In non-medical language, that means cutting down on cholesterol, losing weight, lowering blood pressure, quitting smoking and taking aspirin, the report indicates.

# Thyroid

## Avoid 'natural' thyroid 'health foods', doctors say

There's one "natural" product widely sold in health food stores and by mail that could turn out to be very unhealthy for you, say doctors at Tufts University School of Medicine and the VA Hospital in Boston, Mass. The product to avoid is desiccated thyroid, usually sold in freeze-dried, tablet form, they say.

These doctors refer to a case in which a man with thyroid imbalances tried several times to treat himself with the health-store tablets, according to their report in *Archives of Internal Medicine* (149,9:2117). He took two different "natural" thyroid preparations during a time he was under treatment for problems caused by Graves' disease (old-fashioned goiter, now known as hyperthyroidism). He had had his thyroid gland partially removed years before.

When he finally told his doctors that he was treating himself with the health store tablets at the same time they were trying to treat him with a thyroid hormone, he had a high heart rate, weight loss and unbalanced hormone levels. Those are symptoms of too much thyroid hormones in the blood.

Doctors analyzed the store product that had advertised itself to be free of thyroxine, a thyroid hormone that's also used by doctors to treat thyroid problems. "Despite the disclaimer, the preparation we studied does indeed contain thyroxine and can cause hyperthyroidism if taken in excess," doctors C.T Sawin and Maria H. London write. Too much thyroid hormone can poison you, leading to seizures, heart attack or death, the doctors warn.

They criticize the lack of controls for making and selling "such an unstandard, biologically active product." Many things sold as "health food products" are okay, the doctors say. "Except for the thyroid preparations, none are likely to cause harm, except for their cost. The thyroid products are another matter." They recommend that you steer clear of such products, usually made from ground-up cows' glands. Some health store thyroid tablets include tissue from cow ovaries, bull testes, pancreas, prostate, liver, heart and intestines, says the *Archives* report. Since such tablets are neither drug nor food, there are no government regulations that require minimum standards for content or purity.

Ironically, most such health food store thyroid tablets cost more per tablet than prescription doses of thyroid hormones bought at your pharmacy, the report says.

# Urinary Problems

## Viruses from public restrooms

You were right to be concerned about the hygiene of public toilet seats, according to new research from the University of Arizona.

Normal flushing splatters virus-infected water from the bowl onto the seat, handle and surrounding area, says a report in *American Family Physician* (39,6:20). A microbiologist proved the germ splatter by using time-lapse photography, the report says.

What's the worst area for viruses? The middle stall is used most often, thus receiving the most splatters, the report says.

## Cranberry juice may be a weapon against urinary infections

Does cranberry juice prevent or fight urinary tract infections? Several clinical studies suggest that drinking the sweetened juice of the otherwise bitter berry may cause two changes in the body. The two beneficial changes help in the fight against infections in the pipeline from the kidneys through the bladder.

In one study, reported in *U.S. Pharmacist* (14,5:35), 60 people with urinary infections drank a pint of cranberry juice each day for 21 days. Otherwise, they took no special medications. More than half showed a significant improvement. Two out of 10 were slightly better, and about three out of 10 showed no improvement. In addition, six weeks after they all stopped drinking the juice, more than half those who showed some improvement came down with another urinary infection.

Two other studies reported in the journal also showed some benefits after people drank the juice.

Researchers think the juice raises the acid level of urine, causing it to become hostile to germs. They also think the fructose (a kind of sugar) used to sweeten the juice somehow makes mucous tissue inside the urinary system "slippery" to bacteria—the germs can't grab onto body tissue and multiply.

# Vitamins and Minerals

## Can vitamin and mineral supplements make you smarter?

We've often been told that we "are what we eat," but a new study takes that a step further. It suggests that our intelligence level may be linked to adequate amounts of vitamins and minerals.

In just one school year, tests on 90 high school students in Britain showed an increase in IQ scores in children taking nutritional supplements. Children taking a placebo (a harmless, fake drug) and children not taking anything were used for comparison. Yet, the children receiving the supplements had a marked difference in their non-verbal IQ scores, according to *The Lancet*, a British medical journal.

Nutritionists know which vitamins and minerals aid development in different parts of our brain and body. Yet most believed that people in Western countries received adequate amounts of the necessary vitamins and minerals through their everyday diet.

This is the first study that has been able to document changes in intelligence based on vitamin and mineral supplementation, in people who were not technically deficient. David Benton, who conducted the study, considers the results preliminary. But if you want to start taking more vitamins and minerals, you should use supplements that contain them in the ratios set by the U.S. government and known as the Recommended Dietary Allowance (R.D.A.).

## Magnesium: an overlooked 'miracle' mineral?

You are probably one of the eight of every ten Americans with a significant deficiency in the "trace" mineral, magnesium. And because, as an average American, you consume only about 40 percent of the daily amount of magnesium you need, you may be subjecting yourself to higher risks of high blood pressure, diabetes, pregnancy problems in women, and cardiovascular disease, including abnormal heart rhythms, according to *Science News* (133:356).

Other studies link magnesium deficiency with increased cancer risks, especially esophageal cancer, reports *Maximum Immunity* (pg. 123-4). Recent research showed abnormally low levels of magnesium in the heart muscles of victims of sudden death from heart attacks, indicating that magnesium plays a hitherto unsuspected role in preventing or lessening the effects of heart disease, says *Popular Nutritional Practices* (pg. 226-8).

The further good news about this "miracle" mineral is that recent studies involving humans and animals demonstrated that magnesium-spiked diets decreased the bad effects of pulmonary (lung) high blood pressure, lowered blood cholesterol levels by more than one-third, dramatically reduced migraines and high blood pressure associated with pregnancies, and even prevented the formation of high blood pressure in rats that had been specially treated to make their blood pressure rise.

In another study, researchers found that intravenous solutions of magnesium given to victims immediately after severe heart attacks cut their post-attack death rate in half in the critical four weeks following the attacks, when compared to victims who received only IVs without the added magnesium.

The studies strongly suggest that all of us need to take another look at this little-known "trace" element. While it's been heralded in recent years as an anti-stress mineral, it may be much more important than we realized for maintaining cardiovascular health and for preventing other serious problems, including cancer and high blood pressure.

Because most people don't get even half as much magnesium as they need daily, according to studies presented at the 22nd annual Conference on Trace Substances in Environmental Health and reported in *SN*, "many people face serious consequences—including death—from preventable magnesium deficiency ..., and contributing to the problem is that this deficiency 'is likely to be silent until it is severe,'" according to Mildred S. Seelig, executive director of the American

College of Nutrition in Scarsdale, N.Y.

The studies show that higher levels of dietary magnesium not only prevent development of several serious health problems, but also play a definite role in fighting the bad effects of high blood pressure and fat-rich diets.

For example, in animal tests, results showed that salt-induced hypertension was actually prevented by adding to drinking water four to eight times the recommended daily allowances of the mineral. In another test, rats getting increased magnesium showed few of the ill effects of high blood pressure, induced chemically in their lungs, while rats without the added mineral tripled their lung pressures, doubled their heart sizes, and suffered three to seven-fold thickening of artery walls with corresponding shrinkages of arterial diameters, the report said.

In still another test, this time with rabbits on "normal" cholesterol diets, the researchers showed that increasing magnesium levels to about five times recommended daily allowances resulted in 30 to 40 percent reductions in blood levels of cholesterols and other lipids, when compared to low-magnesium diets. Equally significant, rabbits on high cholesterol diets got megadose magnesium and cut their blood lipid levels by more than half, the study showed. (Lipids are fats or fat-like materials.)

Migraine headaches and high blood pressure, both problems for many pregnant women, are directly linked to inadequate magnesium levels, according to an East Tennessee State University researcher in a report to the same conference. Low magnesium levels also may contribute to stillbirths, miscarriages, and low-birthweight babies, studies with both humans and animals showed. Magnesium supplements greatly reduced such problems, the report said.

While experts believe more than eight of every ten Americans don't get enough magnesium, the highest risk persons are alcoholics and those taking "water pills" (diuretics), digitalis and other heart drugs, and some antibiotics and anti-cancer drugs, according to Seelig. These substances "bind" with magnesium, prevent its absorption into the body, and speed it through the body without letting it have its good effects. Such persons need to check with their doctors about getting a special higher daily supplement of magnesium, the studies suggested.

Soft drink fans also may cut down their magnesium absorption to harmful levels because of the "binding" effect of the phosphates contained in most sodas. For example, a regular 12-ounce soft drink may bind up to 30 milligrams of magnesium and flush it out of the body before it can do its good work.

The recommended dietary allowance (RDA) of magnesium is 350 milligrams for males over 50 and 280 milligrams for females. The RDA for pregnant women and lactating (milk-producing) mothers is even higher — up to 355 milligrams, according to the RDA published by the National Research Council (1985). Three or four soft drinks a day could cause significant deficiencies in magnesium absorption, even in those few people who take enough of the mineral every day.

Good dietary sources of magnesium are leafy dark-green vegetables, whole-grain cereals, figs, lemons, grapefruit, yellow corn, almonds and other nuts and seeds, apples, and seafoods.

However, experts say it's hard to get enough of the mineral just by eating the right foods. They suggest that everyone consider taking a daily supplement in tablet form. One researcher said magnesium would be the one supplement he would recommend for everyone.

You should take magnesium in equal amounts with calcium, several studies said. It can also be bought as magnesium oxide (you get 150 milligrams of magnesium from one 250 milligram tablet of magnesium oxide). It's commonly available in tablets of 133.3 milligrams and may be taken four times a day. Take between meals because magnesium neutralizes stomach acid (remember milk of magnesia?) and acts like an antacid.

Few studies show any poisonous effects of higher-than-RDA doses of magnesium. Experts suggest no more than 3,000 milligrams per day for patients who suffer kidney disfunctions. One study suggested huge doses of the mineral could be linked to excessively low blood pressure and depressed breathing in a few cases. Any long-term use of magnesium in megadoses should, of course, be done only with your doctor's knowledge and permission.

Strong indications are that you will be seeing much more in the near future about this overlooked "miracle" mineral.

In summary, magnesium has been shown in recent studies to do the following:

- Prevent formation of salt-induced high blood pressure
- Cut blood cholesterol levels by more than one-third
- Stop migraines in pregnant women

- Cut death rates in half for post-heart-attack patients
- Prevent formation of several forms of cancer
- Increase oxygen use by muscles, leading to better fitness
- Regulate body's blood sugar metabolism, raising energy level
- Fight depression and act with calcium as a natural tranquilizer
- Help prevent heart attacks
- Aid in stopping calcium deposits, kidney stones, and gallstones
- Keep teeth healthier

## Needed: more of that other 'M' mineral

Most of us need more of another "trace" mineral: manganese. It's an important fighter against osteoporosis (dangerous bone loss among older persons, especially women over 50). It also acts like a traffic cop to insulin, signaling how much to produce and when to release it into the bloodstream, and helps heal tissue damage caused by ozone and other environmental pollutants.

Studies reported in *Science News* (130:199) indicate the body has trouble absorbing manganese even when we eat enough of the right foods. Further, even the recommended dietary allowance (RDA) of 2.5 to 5.0 milligrams per day may be too low. A University of Texas research project involving tests on people showed that one must eat at least 3.8 milligrams each day to keep from running low on the mineral.

The problem is that other ingredients in manganese-rich

foods—like spinach, wheat bran, and tea—cause the mineral to slip through the digestive tract without much of it being absorbed. The manganese present in meats, milk, and eggs, though in smaller amounts than in other foods, is more easily absorbed, which makes these "bio-available" sources of the mineral more important in a nutritious diet.

A better approach may be to take manganese supplements in the form of daily tablets, but watch when you take it and with what other minerals. Studies show that mineral supplements containing iron, calcium, and magnesium cut down on the body's absorption of manganese. So if you take manganese, for best effect, wait several hours before taking other kinds of mineral tablets.

The tip-off to the link between bone problems and manganese deficiency occurred to biologist Paul Saltman after he studied the chronic bone fractures suffered by basketball superstar Bill Walton. X-rays showed Walton had a form of osteoporosis, resulting in continuous bone loss and breakage. Blood tests showed the athlete had no manganese and half the normal levels of zinc and copper. The researcher took Walton off his macrobiotic diet and put him on mineral supplements, and within six weeks Walton resumed his career playing basketball.

The mineral plays an important role in helping specialized cells break down old bone tissue and replace it with new bone cells. A manganese deficiency weakens the bone-building cells, resulting in increasingly porous bones and symptoms of osteoporosis, the report said. Another study of Belgium women with severe osteoporosis showed the women had one-fourth the manganese levels in their blood as women of the same age without the bone disease.

The moral of the story is clear: supplement your diet with manganese, being careful not to take it with blocking agents like magnesium, iron, calcium, phytate and fiber in bran, oxalic acid in things like spinach, and tannins in tea.

## Confusion may mean a nutritional deficiency

It's considered a medical emergency. Doctors see signs of mental confusion, verbal nonsense, wobbly walk, uncoordinated movements and eyesight disturbances in people with a severe deficiency of vitamin B1, also called thiamine.

"The age-old and potentially fatal nutritional deficiency ... requires immediate thiamine (B1) replacement to ensure the best long-term outcome," says an article in *Emergency Medicine* (21,7:13). "Withholding treatment for only a few hours from patients you may think have the disease may worsen the prognosis."

The condition, known medically as Wernicke's encephalopathy, can strike not only alcoholics but also people with kidney disease, patients with thyroid gland problems, and compulsive dieters suffering from self-induced starvation, a condition called anorexia nervosa.

While its symptoms are serious, the disease itself "is probably totally reversible if treated early," the report said. Even a previously healthy person can drain her body's entire supply of thiamine within three weeks, the report warns.

That's especially true if the person is for any reason receiving an intravenous infusion of glucose over a period of several days.

Thiamine is a water-soluble vitamin, the first of the B vitamins to be isolated in its pure form (that's why it's known as B1). Normal levels of thiamine are necessary for converting carbohydrates in food into energy, for the proper operation of the nervous system, and for growth and repair of body tissues. Thiamine is found naturally in yeast, liver, whole-grain products, wheat, eggs, milk, nuts, potatoes, leafy green vegetables, kidney beans, and seeds.

"The need for thiamine is increased when carbohydrate consumption is high," according to *Vitamin and Mineral Encyclopedia* (FC&A Publishing, 1987: p. 92). Exercise or emotional stress may increase the energy needs of the body and the body's need for thiamine. More thiamine is needed in pregnancy, during breast-feeding, when fever is present, during and after surgery, and in cases of hyperthyroidism.

Other things that deplete thiamine include sulfa drugs, oral contraceptives and estrogen hormone treatments, air pollution and certain food additives like nitrates and sulfates.

Adult men normally need about 1.5 milligrams of thiamine each day. Adult women need somewhat less, about 1.1 milligrams. However, if special conditions warrant, as listed above, your regular thiamine intake may need to be supplemented.

Always be sure to ask your doctor or healthcare provider about supplements, however, because certain people should not take thiamine. For diabetics, for example, thiamine supplements can interfere with insulin levels in the blood.

# An internal insect repellent?

Taking vitamin B1 supplements, known as thiamine, may provide a natural repellent against insects.

In a small study at Michigan's Lake Superior State College, thiamine supplements seemed to protect volunteers from mosquito bites. Students took the supplement or a placebo (a fake supplement) immediately before they went out into the woods and then kept track of the number of mosquito bites they received.

There were fewer mosquito bites on people who took the thiamine, and now researchers are trying to duplicate the study with more people, to confirm the results.

# Zinc can help you live longer

Low levels of zinc can reduce your body's immune response and increase your risk of infections. But too much zinc can reduce the effectiveness of copper, iron and other minerals in your system.

A recent study in *Journal of Nutrition for the Elderly* (8,1:3) indicates that the RDA (or recommended dietary allowance) provides enough zinc to keep a normal person's immune system responding well without harming the needed absorption of other minerals.

Adults should get 15 milligrams of zinc daily, the RDA according to the federal government. Liver, seafood (especially herring and shellfish), dairy products, meat, whole grains and eggs are good sources of zinc, while vegetables are poor sources of zinc.

Adequate zinc consumption may actually help to lower death rates. That's because a less healthy immune system results in more infections among elderly people. And more infections result in higher death rates for seniors.

In tests in hospital patients, people with healing problems like leg ulcers or pressure sores also had the lowest levels of zinc in their bodies, reports the *British Journal of Nutrition* (59,2:181).

Zinc also may help prevent "macular degeneration," a deterioration of the nerves in the eyes. In a study at the Louisiana State University Eye Center, older adults who took zinc supplements for up to two years had less eye deterioration than people who didn't receive the supplements.

In addition, zinc also has been reported to help fight cancer and skin disease, to improve the sense of taste, and to shorten the length of the common cold, says the *Journal of Nutrition for the Elderly* (8,2:49).

Aging alone does not cause low levels of zinc, according to *American Journal of Clinical Nutrition* (48,2:343). Since many elderly people reduce their food intake, researchers believe that older people, especially those in institutions, are not usually getting the minimum daily requirement for zinc. A study at Bowling Green State University found that "dietary zinc intakes were inadequate in 67 percent" of the elderly.

The journal *Human Nutrition and Applied Nutrition* (40,6:440) reports that in one acute medical care ward studied, the meals served by the institution provided only about one-half the RDA of zinc — even if the patient ate everything on the plate!

Phytic acid, found in grains and other dietary fiber, interferes with the absorption of zinc, so people on high fiber or vegetarian diets may not get adequate amounts of zinc.

Normal cooking "decreases the phytic acid content and improves zinc absorption," says the *Journal of Nutrition* (117,11:1898).

Zinc supplements above the RDA interfere with the body's metabolism of copper and iron. "Many women might be at risk for iron deficiency" even with supplements of less than four times the RDA of zinc, says the *American Journal of Clinical Nutrition* (49,1:145).

Decreased levels of copper, which helps in the formation of bone, hair and skin and is important in the formation of hemoglobin and red blood cells, are also caused by excessive doses of zinc supplements.

While the proper amount of zinc greatly helps the body's immune system, too much zinc has the opposite effect. Excessive intake of zinc is suspected to impair the immune system's response, says the *Journal of the American Medical Association* (252,11:1443). Too much zinc also lowers the level of "good" cholesterol known as HDL, according to *Metabolism* (34:519).

Consuming the RDA of zinc is essential for good health. But high doses should be avoided because of its effects on other minerals and because of possible negative effects on cholesterol levels and the immune system.

# Vitamin stories

Your arteries may need more vitamin C than current government guidelines call for, according to a report in *Science News* (136,9:133).

Scientists at the University of California at Berkeley are calling for an increase in the recommended daily allowance of vitamin C, after studies there showed that vitamin C neutralizes toxic chemicals in the blood that initiate hardening of the arteries.

The chemicals, called free radicals, damage low-density lipoproteins ("bad" cholesterol, as you may remember) and set off a chain reaction that leads to clogged arteries.

Vitamin C "disarms" free radicals, these researchers say.

"I was quite surprised at how much better a scavenger of free radicals [vitamin C] was, especially when compared to vitamin E," says biochemist Balz Frei.

Vitamin C performed even better than naturally occurring substances in the blood that fight toxic intruders, the report says.

Elderly Americans, especially those who are bedridden, may need higher amounts of vitamin D to prevent rickets-like disease, according to a report in *Drug Therapy* (19,8:63).

Studies suggest that with increasing age, the skin cannot produce vitamin D efficiently. In addition, the intestines cannot effectively absorb supplements, the report says.

Sun exposure increases vitamin D production in the body, but in one study, even people living in sunny climates had lower vitamin D levels.

Daily 5- to 15-milligram supplements of folic acid appear safe for healthy people, according to a report in the *American Journal of Clinical Nutrition* (50,2:353).

Folic acid, one of eight vitamins in the vitamin B complex, is vital to red blood cell production. It is found in medications used to treat everything from psoriasis to AIDS.

Scientists say more studies are needed to determine whether folic acid supplements cause toxicity in these patients or decrease a medication's effectiveness.

Folic acid overdose may mask symptoms of severe anemia and interfere with zinc absorption. Pregnant women taking supplements should be sure to get enough zinc as well.

If you are over 50, you may be short-changing yourself on vitamin B6, suggests a report in *The American Journal of Clinical Nutrition* (50,2:391).

Recommended daily allowances (RDAs) of vitamins and minerals are based on the needs of young, healthy adults, say Danish researchers.

The current RDA for B6 is 2.0 milligrams for men and 1.6 milligrams for women.

The researchers suggest that RDAs for the elderly be based on the older person's individual needs.

Those needs likely are different from those of a young person.

The scientists are concerned specifically about vitamin B6, the levels of which decrease in the body with increasing age, sometimes leading to a deficiency.

Vitamin B6 promotes healthy skin, red blood cells and teeth and gums.

Researchers encourage older people to eat more fruits,

vegetables and potatoes.

A carefully balanced, healthful diet usually ensures the right amount of B6 and other vitamins.

But people who don't get enough nutrition from their regular diets may need vitamin B6 supplements, the report says.

# Not enough copper and vitamin E in RDA?

While recent changes to the government's official vitamin and mineral recommendations add two nutrients — vitamin K and selenium — and cut back on recommended levels of several others, some researchers worry that most of us may not get nearly enough of two other nutrients. Of course, check with your doctor before taking any supplements.

One of the deficiencies may be vitamin E, says William A. Pryor of Louisiana State University.

Several studies now suggest that we may need to take up to 10 times the current RDA for vitamin E, argues Pryor in *Science News* (136,18:277).

Pryor says the vitamin is harmless even at 50 times the current RDA. He reasons that taking more E couldn't hurt and might help.

However, one study suggested that people who take high doses of vitamin E have higher death rates than those on smaller doses.

The new RDA is unchanged — 10 milligrams for adult males and 8 milligrams for adult females. Vitamin E is the body's hardest-working anti-oxidant, meaning that it attacks and neutralizes harmful chemical combinations in the blood and tissues. There's strong evidence that it blocks tumor growth and cancer spread.

The other nutrient shortage may be copper, which doesn't even have an official RDA, according to Leslie M. Klevay, a scientist at the U.S. Agriculture Department's nutrition research center in Grand Forks, N.D.

Klevay says that half the U.S. population gets less than 1.5 milligrams of copper daily. That's half what is loosely suggested by the National Research Council. More worrisome — one-third of all Americans get less than one milligram of copper daily.

Studies have shown that a copper shortage that severe can cause dozens of body changes linked to heart disease, including high cholesterol and high blood pressure, the report says.

# Weight Loss

## Being overweight can hurt your chances for a long and healthy life

In addition to detracting from your appearance, being more than 15 percent overweight can lead to many health problems including joint disease, coronary artery disease, stroke, high blood pressure, high cholesterol levels, diabetes, gallstones, gouty arthritis, osteoarthritis, cancer, skin problems, breathing difficulties, sleep apnea, kidney disease, increased risk during surgery, increased risk of complications during pregnancy, and a delay in the discovery of abdominal diseases. It also leads to — believe it or not — traffic accidents, according to a report in the *American Journal of Clinical Nutrition* (49,5:993).

Having more than one risk factor raises your chances of becoming ill. For example, high blood pressure increases your stroke and heart-disease risk; smoking increases your heart-disease risk even more. If you're overweight, add diabetes to the list and raise the odds on the other two diseases.

"On the whole, diet plays a very important part in the development of [heart disease], cancer and diabetes," according to the report. One last reminder: "[Diet] becomes even more meaningful if the harmful effects of heavy alcohol drinking are taken into account."

## Weight loss: your sex and age are a factor

Weight loss is guilty of both age and sex discrimination. That's the finding announced by the Centers for Disease Control in Atlanta, a federal health agency. Young women gain more weight than young men, but older women lose more weight than older men, according to the new CDC study.

Due to reduced physical activity and other lifestyle changes beginning in early adulthood, men and women between ages 25 and 34 are likely to gain an average of seven pounds over their next 10 years.

But the CDC research shows that just over six percent of adults in that age group will gain nearly 30 pounds in the same period — putting them at substantially greater risk of high cholesterol, high blood pressure and heart disease.

Younger women are more likely than men of the same age bracket to add extra weight. The average American male can expect to pick up an additional six pounds between his 25th and 35th birthdays. But the average woman will gain even more during that same decade— about seven and three-quarters pounds. And while about 4 percent of the younger men will gain more than 30 pounds in 10 years, women of the same age are nearly twice as likely to gain this much excess weight, the CDC reports.

In the first nationwide study of its kind, investigators from the CDC analyzed data on 9,897 adults aged 25 to 74. Each person's weight was recorded twice over a 10-year period. Nearly 13 percent of the adults 25-34 in the study, who had started with normal weights, had become overweight 10 years later.

Researchers found that the average adult tends to gain weight until about age 55, regardless of the sex of the individual — but the incidence of major weight gain is roughly twice as high for women as it is for men. Interestingly, it was the skinny guys who were most likely to put on added pounds. "The men in the study who were underweight during their first weighing had the highest risk of major weight gain," according to the report.

However, among women, the ones who were fat just got fatter. Women who were overweight at the first weighing had the highest risk of major weight gain over the next decade.

In the study, a 20 percent increase in body weight was considered a major weight gain. In other words, a man who weighed 175 pounds in the first weighing period and then put on 35 pounds over the next 10 years would qualify as a "major" weight gainer in the study.

"After age 55, however, both men and women tend to lose weight," said CDC study director David Williamson. "We found that individuals lose an average of two to 10 pounds between the ages of 55 and 64, but in this age group, women actually lose more weight than men. For some reason, women seem to be more extreme in both trends."

The CDC researchers believe that the weight gain experienced by most younger adults is potentially hazardous to health, even if it doesn't lead to obesity. "Most of the weight being gained by younger adults is in the form of fat, not muscle," Williamson warned. "We want to emphasize that the process of gaining weight can increase the likelihood of high cholesterol levels or high blood pressure, even if you aren't classed as obese."

Physical activity needs more emphasis in weight control, and diet alone is seldom enough, according to the investigators. "The weight gain that begins in early adulthood may be a direct result of changes in the average person's exercise habits," Williamson said. "Teenagers typically are very active, but physical activity often tapers off in adulthood."

The best time to deal with the problems of body fat and being overweight is before they occur, Williamson stressed, "because, as anyone knows who's ever tried it, it's very difficult to lose weight once you've gained it. It may be easier to keep it off in the first place."

## The danger of yo-yo dieting

The more often you diet, the harder it is for you to lose weight, a new study reports. Not only that, but there's a danger to on-again-off-again dieting. Losing weight quickly, then gaining it right back, may increase your risk of sudden death from heart disease, according to a new study by researchers at Northwestern University.

"Men who showed the greatest up-and-down weight swings also had the highest risk of sudden death from coronary heart disease," says weight loss expert Dr. Kelly Brownell of the University of Pennsylvania School of Medicine.

Weight loss and weight gain, known as weight cycles or yo-yo dieting, is a way of life for many people. However, researchers are discovering that yo-yo dieting may be more harmful than not losing weight at all.

Here are some of the pitfalls of yo-yo dieting:

(1) It may slow your body's metabolism and make it more difficult for you to lose the weight again. Studies on animals by Dr. Per Bjorntorp of Sweden found that losing and regaining weight greatly increases "food efficiency." The report in *American Journal of Clinical Nutrition* (36,3: 444) defines food efficiency as how much weight is gained compared to the amount of calories that are consumed. Only if someone was facing starvation would this natural defense mechanism be helpful. Under normal circumstances, "increased food efficiency" simply makes dieting more difficult.

In *Physiological Behavior* ( 38,4: 459), Brownell explains, "frequent dieting may make subsequent weight loss more difficult." In his study, animals that went through two cycles of weight loss and weight gain, "showed significant increases in food efficiency" in the second weight loss/weight gain period. "Weight loss occurred at half the rate and regain at three times the rate in the second cycle .... At the end of the experiment, cycled animals had a four-fold increase in food efficiency compared to obese animals of the same weight who had not cycled." The tests show, in other words, for every new weight-loss diet you try, it's likely you'll lose weight more slowly and regain it more quickly.

If your diet is successful and you do lose weight, you'll have to eat a lot less from now on than you're used to eating. Tests by Dr. Jules Hirsch of Rockefeller University in New York reported in *Metabolism* (33,2:164) also show that obese people who have lost weight on a diet require less energy (or calories) to maintain their body weight.

"In order to maintain a reduced weight, some reduced-obese ... patients must restrict their food intake to approximately 25 percent less than" what would be expected for their new, lighter body size, Hirsch says.

(2) Yo-yo dieting usually shifts weight from your hips and thighs to your stomach, where it is more dangerous to your health. A fat stomach or waist is linked to an increased risk of stroke in men and higher rates of heart failure in both sexes, according to researchers from Boston University, reports *Natural Healing News* (1,2:1).

(3) Yo-yo dieting actually may increase your desire for fatty foods. Studies by Reed and Rodin, reported in *Physiological Behavior* (42,4:389), found that animals on a severely restricted diet chose more fatty foods once they were taken off the diet. Since fatty foods are less healthy for us, an increased desire for fats "may have negative health consequences."

(4) Yo-yo dieting may increase your body's proportion of

fat to lean tissue. According to Brownell's Weight Cycling Project, when people lose a lot of weight by dieting — especially on crash diets or low-protein diets — they lose muscle tissue along with the fat. However, when they regain the weight, the addition usually comes back as fat, not as muscle, Brownell says.

This is a good reason to combine diet with exercise — exercise will help you to lose fat and not muscle so you'll be less likely to gain the weight back. "The addition of exercise in the diet treatment did show an effect in weight and fat loss," reports the *American Journal of Clinical Nutrition* (49,3:409).

Yo-yo dieting strains your body and increases your risk of sudden death from heart disease. But for many people, a permanent weight reduction is a good thing. The point is to keep the weight off once you lose it. That may mean eating about one-fourth less calories from now on — a permanent diet, instead of a yo-yo diet.

Before going on any diet, check with your physician first. And be sure to work with your doctor or healthcare provider to discover a safe weight-loss and weight maintenance program that you can follow — from now on.

## Learn to suppress your appetite naturally

If overeating is your problem, you can learn these tricks to suppress your appetite and control your weight.

Drink a glass of grapefruit juice, tomato juice, or unsweetened lemonade as an appetizer about 20 minutes before you eat. The acid in the juice and the volume of fluid that you drink will help you feel full, and you will be able to eat less.

Throughout the day, you can drink lemon-water as a natural appetite suppressant. Just add the freshly-squeezed juice from a lemon to a glass of water. Slowly sip on this drink throughout the day. Drinking just two glasses of lemon-water a day will help you control your appetite.

Place a bottle of mouthwash in front of your refrigerator door, suggests the Good Wellness Program for Weight Management. If you stray into the kitchen looking for "something to eat," you will have to move the mouthwash first. Use the mouthwash before taking anything out of the fridge. Rinsing with the mouthwash may help satisfy the cravings without consuming any calories.

Try squeezing your earlobe for 60 seconds before you eat. This is an ancient technique of acupressure that may help curb your appetite.

Also, be sure to eat slowly. Put your utensils down after each bite. It takes several minutes for the stomach to tell the brain that it is full. Eating slowly will help you realize you're full before you overeat.

## Lose weight by changing when you eat

How about a diet that lets you eat everything you're eating now but you'll lose weight? Would you try it?

Most people can shed unwanted pounds by changing the

time of day they eat, according to *Postgraduate Medicine* (79:4,352). Eating earlier in the day could let you lose as much as 10 pounds in a month. More than 600 volunteers lost between five and 10 pounds each in one month, Tulane University researchers discovered. The participants didn't change what they ate, *just the time of day* it was eaten.

Breakfast and lunch became the main meals of the day, with only a light snack in the afternoon. People in the study could not go to bed at night within eight hours of their last meal. The researchers speculate that eating the major part of our daily calories early in the day allows the food to be used to produce energy; therefore, fewer calories are left over to change into fat.

Even dieting is more effective when the calories are consumed earlier in the day, a study by Dr. Frank Halberg, at the University of Minnesota confirmed. People on 2,000 calories per day diets lost 2.2 pounds per week if they ate all 2,000 calories at breakfast. But people who ate the 2,000 calories at dinner gained weight or lost very little.

## How you sleep can affect your weight

Sleeping in a cold room can increase weight loss, reports *Harper's Bazaar*. Just as exercise helps burn off calories, having your body maintain its normal temperature will help you lose weight while you're sleeping. Helping your body to "exercise" during a comfortable sleep cannot be considered a rapid diet technique, but in the long run, it can help burn off unwanted calories.

A cool room at night with fresh air circulating is also thought to contribute to a good night's sleep.

## Rapid weight loss may trigger formation of gallstones

Drastic dieting to cause rapid weight loss in fat people may lead to increased formation of painful gallstones, a new medical study suggests. Doctors found a big increase in gallstone formation among 51 obese people who participated in an 8-week quick weight-loss program, compared to a group of overweight people who didn't diet.

In fact, one out of every four people on the crash diet developed gallstones, according to the report in *Archives of Internal Medicine* (149,8:1750). In all, 13 of the 51 men and women developed the hard cholesterol-containing stones during the 8-week diet. Three of them required gallbladder-removal surgery within a few weeks of quitting the diet. A control group of non-dieting fat people, on the other hand, showed no abnormal gallbladder developments, the report says.

"A large number of individuals undergoing prolonged calorie restriction and rapid weight loss may be at risk for development of gallstones," the doctors report.

The dieters ranged in age from 27 to 58, and all were more than 30 percent over ideal weights. They went on a 500-calorie-per-day diet. A normal intake can range from 1,200 to

2,000 calories per day. Average weight loss was between 36 and 39 pounds per person. The ones who developed gallstones, on average, lost about three pounds more than the ones who remained free of cholesterol sludge or stones in the gallbladder.

Obesity itself is a big risk for developing gallstones. Out of every 10 greatly overweight people, three to five of them eventually develop the cholesterol stones, the report says. A study in the *New England Journal of Medicine* (321,9:563) found that "grossly overweight" women are six times more likely to develop gallstones, compared to women whose weight is average for their height. Even "slightly overweight" women face nearly double the risk of developing gallstones, the *NEJM* report says.

Not all gallstones are formed from cholesterol, and not all of them cause trouble. But when they plug up bile ducts, they trigger pain, swelling, jaundice (yellowing of the skin) and other problems, sometimes requiring surgery. Some drugs and treatments can slow stone formation or dissolve gallstones already formed.

The doctors in the *Archives* study theorize that sudden, drastic dieting causes the liver to churn out bile that's overloaded with cholesterol, leading to the formation of gallstones.

The doctors still think fat people should lose weight, since obesity is a major health risk for heart disease, high blood pressure and diabetes. Using stone-dissolving treatments along with a slowed-down weight loss plan may reduce the risk of gallstone formation, the report says.

If you want to lose weight fast with a low-calorie diet,

check with your doctor first about the relative risks involved, the researchers suggest.

# Caution on the "grapefruit diet"

It took three months of vitamin and mineral treatment to pull a 47-year-old New York woman out of a diet-caused nose dive into anemia, fatigue, leg swelling and abdominal pains and bloating.

She had used the so-called grapefruit diet for two years and had lost about 50 pounds, but her health had faded during the process, according to a doctor's report in *The Journal of the American Board of Family Practice* (2,2:130).

She had been eating unrestricted breakfasts, dinners and snacks but nothing at lunch but a grapefruit.

Her doctor found that she suffered from an iron deficiency, causing anemia, and a severe case of vitamin B12 shortage. The doctor put the woman in the hospital and gave her a red cell transfusion to beef up her blood.

For the next three months, the doctor put the woman on a regular nutritional scheme with the addition of a multivitamin supplement, one milligram of folic acid by mouth daily, iron sulfate by mouth twice a day, and monthly injections of B12.

A year later, the woman was still eating balanced normal nutritious meals, had regained her energy and had kept her weight to within five pounds of what she weighed when she first saw the doctor, the report said. What she discarded, the doctor said, was the grapefruit diet.

# 9 D's of Dieting

If you aren't trying to lose weight, but the pounds are dropping off nonetheless, should you be concerned?

Yes, doctors say, if you've lost 5 percent of your normal body weight over the last year.

You should check with your doctor, for example, if you are a 170-lb. man who's lost 10 pounds, or a 125-lb. woman who's lost six and a half pounds unexpectedly.

But before you go, you can help your doctor by taking a look at the major causes of weight loss in the elderly, according to a recent outline in *Geriatrics* (44,4:31).

If you are having any of these problems — called the nine Ds of elderly weight loss — tell your doctor.

The more information you can provide, the less time and money you will spend on unnecessary tests to find the cause of your weight loss.

• **Dentition.** This is a fancy word for dentures and teeth. Poorly fitting dentures may make chewing painful and eating a less pleasurable activity.

Always clean your dentures well; "dirty dentures" may affect taste.

Gum disease also affects taste, so regular dental checkups are in order, even if you wear dentures.

• **Disease.** Some diseases, such as heart disease and

cancer, sap the body's strength and may lead to weight loss.

If you have such an illness, talk to your doctor about what you can do to keep up your appetite.

• **Dysgeusia**. Another fancy term, this means that as you age, your ability to taste and smell diminishes, which in turn takes the pleasures out of eating.

Certain drugs, such as theophylline, may add to the problem.

Try adding more herbs and spices to your food.

• **Depression**. This is one of the most common causes of elderly weight loss and affects one in 10 older Americans.

Lifestyle changes, such as retirement, loss of a spouse and health or financial problems, may trigger depression.

Once you recognize depression, however, it can be treated.

• **Diarrhea**. People who suffer from diarrhea usually eat less to avoid it.

But you should know that diarrhea itself is not a cause of weight loss.

It is a symptom of another condition, and once it's treated, your appetite should return.

• **Dysphagia**. This means difficulty in swallowing, coughing or sneezing.

People with nervous disorders such as Parkinson's disease often have dysphagia.

Some may have the sensation of food sticking in their

throat. The condition is treatable.

• **Dementia.** People suffering from dementia, such as Alzheimer's patients, are not able to watch their food and beverage intake and may go hungry and thirsty.

They may not enjoy eating and have trouble swallowing. These people need assistance when dining.

• **Dysfunction.** This describes the social causes of weight loss:

An elderly widower who never learned to cook for himself; a widow trying to save money; elderly people who have no transportation to the grocery store or who fear walking on icy sidewalks or in dangerous neighborhoods.

• **Drugs.** Antidepressants and diuretics, among others, "may cause dry mouth, which interferes with taste and swallowing."

Others, such as theophylline, may cause stomach upset. Still others affect the taste and smell.

If you are taking medication, ask your doctor about its side effects.

# The power of prayer:
# concluding remarks

The secrets in this book are based on medical reports of natural healing, but don't overlook the <u>supernatural</u> healing power of God. God is our Creator and Master Physician. If you put your faith and trust in God, by following Jesus Christ, we believe that your prayers for healing will be answered according to God's will.

Although God may not answer "yes" to every request, there is ample evidence of the power of prayer that is submissive to God's will.

Not only are there many anecdotal reports of unexplained miracles, but one scientific study has shown that prayers to "the Judeo-Christian God" were effective in treating seriously ill hospital patients.

If you would like to know more about how to know God and have eternal life through a personal relationship with Jesus Christ, please write to FC&A, Dept. JC 90, 103 Clover Green, Peachtree City, Georgia, 30269. We believe getting to know God better will change your life!